PRETTY
ICONIC

fnk

HUGHES

For Marvin and Arthur

This was Mum's Ferraris and Pokémon

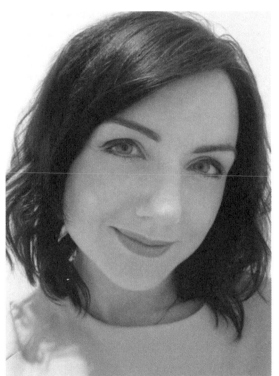

Sali Hughes is a journalist, broadcaster, *Guardian Weekend*, *The Pool* and *Empire* columnist. A former magazine editor, she has written for many publications including *Grazia*, *The Observer*, *Elle*, *The Telegraph*, *Marie Claire*, *Cosmopolitan*, *Vogue*, *Stylist*, *Woman & Home*, *Good Housekeeping* and *Red*, where she is Contributing Editor. She appears frequently on BBC Radio 4 and on Soho Radio, where she hosts her own show and is co-founder of Beauty Banks, a non-profit providing essential toiletries to people living in serious poverty. She lives with her two sons and husband, comedy writer Daniel Maier, in Brighton.

Twitter: @salihughes
Instagram: @salihughes
#PrettyIconic

PRETTY
ICONIC
SALI
HUGHES

a personal look at the
beauty products that
changed the world

Photographs by
Jake Walters

4th ESTATE • *London*

4th Estate
An imprint of HarperCollins*Publishers*
1 London Bridge Street
London SE1 9GF
www.4thEstate.co.uk

This 4th Estate
paperback edition
published 2018

First published in Great Britain
by 4th Estate in 2016

13 5 7 9 8 6 4 2

Text copyright ©
Pretty Honest Ltd 2016

All photographs ©
Jake Walters 2016
www.Jakewalters.com

Illustrations by Mel Elliott
www. ilovemel.me

Design and Art Direction
by BLOK
www.blokdesign.co.uk

Typeset by GS Typesetting

A catalogue record for this book is
available from the British Library.

ISBN 978-0-00-819455-0

Printed and bound in China

MIX
Paper from
responsible sources
FSC   FSC C007454
www.fsc.org

FSC™ is a non-profit international
organisation established to promote
the responsible management of the
world's forests. Products carrying the
FSC label are independently certified to
assure consumers that they come from
forests that are managed to meet the
social, economic and ecological needs
of present and future generations, and
other controlled sources.

Find out more about HarperCollins
and the environment at
www.harpercollins.co.uk/green

In my loft, there's a red plastic B&Q toolbox filled with make-up no longer fit for purpose but that I'll never, ever throw away. There's a dried out, once-black Body Shop eyeliner pen that my mother put in my Christmas stocking circa 1989, which I wore with cut-off Levi's and a lycra bodysuit to Cardiff's Square Club. There's a pot of Clinique face powder in a dreadfully unsuitable shade of pink, that I'd saved at least six weeks' pocket money to buy before realising it made me look embalmed. The Rimmel lilac eye palette I was convinced made me appear 18, the apricot lip balm bought for me by fourth form squeeze Hywel White, a dry, cracked Kryolan professional concealer palette bought in haste less than a year later, when I heard I'd be making up the Pet Shop Boys, the half-used Prescriptives foundation given to me by my boss because I could never have afforded my own, and the Mary Quant eyeshadows I found in a dusty box in a discount chemist on South Molton Street, and thought I'd won the lottery. These aren't just products. This isn't just a toolbox. It's a time capsule, and everything in it takes me back to a moment, a hope, a mistake, an achievement. These unassuming bits and pieces each have their own significance and collectively make something as potent and meaningful as any long-saved C90 compilation. They're my beauty mixtape.

But like any true music lover, I always want to hear something new that excites me just as much. And so it is with beauty. Good job, because I'm sent around 2000 new beauty products a year, from designer fragrances and state of the art skincare, to supermarket shampoos and lipsticks costing less than a two pinter of milk – all of them promising something new and extraordinary. It's an extremely fortunate and wonderful position to be in (teenage me is never far from memory, and believe me, she's having kittens), but not one without some stress. Storage and eating surfaces aside, I worry constantly that I'll miss something wonderful. A product so brilliant, so revolutionary and life-changing, that it will deserve to become a beauty icon, used by millions, remembered always, popped in someone's future treasured toolbox.

But what makes an icon? Quality alone is neither enough nor strictly the point. The beauty products in this book aren't always, in my view, the best – at least not for me personally. Very many of my all time favourites are not here (and as ever, everything in this book has been chosen by me and me alone, with absolutely no commercial consideration). I happen to prefer By Terry Touche Veloutée and Clinique Airbrush Concealer to the mighty YSL Touche Éclat pen, but in terms of influence, memorability and its creation of an entire beauty category, the latter wins by a country mile. Likewise, you may not love Chanel No 5. But the fact is, you will probably still have an opinion on what is, without question, the towering icon of perfumery. You might not find Estée Lauder Advanced Night Repair ideal for your skin but in all likelihood, the serum you *do* love would not exist without it. These three items, in their own ways, changed how countless beauty products were designed and used thereafter. They are reference points, or the stars of a beauty 'moment', or so familiar and relied upon that they're practically part of the family.

While to many, beauty products are silly, an irrelevance, the currency of the vain and the shallow, they are, to me, the furniture of our lives. Just as we chart life's journey through music, food and places, I also attribute the same importance and sentimentality to the beauty products I saw, touched, and smelled all around me. The flipping of a lid on a bottle of Johnson's baby lotion triggers a Proustian rush. I'm immediately back in my grandmother's living room, my clean pyjamas warming on the fireguard, the soothing hum of *Antiques Roadshow* and the rattle of a twin tub washer in the background. I don't just remember my first kiss, I remember the Miss Selfridge Copperknockers lipstick smeared messily over my cheeks afterwards. My first ever gig was notable not only because I saw The Smiths on their last tour, but because I'd stolen my mum's Rimmel lipliner and Givenchy Ysatis perfume for this life-changing occasion. A memorable beauty product can transport me to my nan's backstreet curl and set parlour, my teenage cabin bed, a school disco or my wedding day. When I look back at pivotal moments in my life, I can almost always remember the cosmetics and toiletries that accompanied me, and how I came to be wearing them. These are the lotions, potions, creams, colours and powders that defined how we presented ourselves to the outside world. They were companions at major life events. The perfumes that gave us backbone for important job interviews, the make-up chosen to come on our first dates with a partner, the toiletries taken on family holidays, the little luxury bought with a first pay packet.

It's easy to forget that these cosy, familiar make-up, skincare and toiletries of our youth were often born from world-changing innovation and where particularly interesting, I've tried to provide some context. Likewise, if I feel a product is oft-misunderstood or unfairly maligned, I've suggested best practice techniques and tips, on how better to utilise them. In Future Icons are some products that, to me, represent either an unforgettable moment – welcome or otherwise – or a great advance in beauty. Whether history will agree with me remains to be seen.

Most importantly, I should say that my interpretation of the word 'icon' is wholly subjective and seen very much through the lens of a 41-year-old British woman and is therefore a shamelessly Western view of products. I absolutely acknowledge that Japanese beauty rituals and technology, for just one example, have always been extremely influential and that in recent years, Korean products have changed our beauty culture, but they don't have the same personal meaning to me (no doubt they will to our children). Radox, Poison and Sun-In – these are the products that made *my* life. There will, I hope, be some products you remember from your own upbringing. The shampoo that sat at the corner of your childhood bath, the pot of face cream your mother kept on the bedside table, perhaps. There will no doubt be others that are entirely new to you and equally, some omissions that figure hugely in your past or present but not in my own – I would really love to hear what they are.

THE
ICONS

In perfume-nerd circles, saying Chanel No 5 is your favourite perfume is as obvious and dreary as declaring *Citizen Kane* your favourite film, Shakespeare and the *Mona Lisa* your favourite playwright and painting. But sometimes, things are seen as the best because they simply *are*. There's no use fighting a towering icon just to be contrary and interesting. And even if you don't like No 5 (and very many genuinely don't – smell is a wholly subjective business), you should still respect this remarkable 94-year-old French perfume and what is arguably the most iconic and recognisable beauty product of all time.

No 5 was created by the extraordinarily clever and talented Russian-French perfumer Ernest Beaux, but, for me, his creation is Coco Chanel from crystal stopper to basenote. The couturier had been obsessed with cleanliness from a young age, but was frustrated with the ephemeral characteristics of fresh-smelling citrus colognes. She wanted something stronger, longer lasting, more characterful, and so Beaux mixed traditional floral extracts with aldehydes – isolated chemicals that artificially gave a clean smell, but stuck around on the skin until bedtime. These synthetics were deemed inferior and tacky in 1921, but Coco gave not a damn. Beaux made up ten versions of the scent, numbered 1–5 and 20–24. Superstitious Coco chose five, her lucky number. She packaged it in a typically unfussy flacon, inspired by men's toiletries and adorned with nothing more than a square label and simple type – a pretty subversive move in itself, when luxury perfumes came in big, blowsy balloon-atomisers. The No 5 bottle – since then, the subject of works by artists and photographers such as Andy Warhol, Louis-Nicolas Darbon and Ed Feingersh in his portraits of Marilyn Monroe – is as recognisable a French icon as the Eiffel Tower.

The scent itself – powdery, fizzy, sexy, grown-up, chic and refined – is magnificent, whether or not your particular bag (though impressively, it remains the world's bestselling scent). But for me it goes way beyond smell. It's true to say that outside those with my immediate family, the most enduring relationship of my life has been with No 5. I discovered it at 12 years old and wore it with vintage Levi's and Smiths T-shirts at school discos; I spritzed it over my uniform when I ran away from home three years later. It moved to London with me when I had nothing but a PE bag worth of belongings, it lost my virginity with me, it came on my driving test, it laced my smiley T-shirts and accompanied me to acid house raves (thankfully, not on the same day). Naturally, it was a guest at my wedding. Some years later, broken, confused and tearful, I considered no other fragrance for my father's funeral. On such a hideous and unwanted day, I needed an old friend to stop me from falling.

Nowadays, I don't wear No 5 every day – perhaps once or twice a month. I love perfume too much to be monogamous, and besides, while familiarity could never breed contempt, to use it daily is to forget how wonderful it really is. But when I have a big work day, or special occasion, I unfailingly turn to its strength, unflappable appropriateness (No 5 is literally never a bad idea), respect for occasion and soft, welcoming femininity. I call No 5 my backbone in a bottle, the loaded pistol in my knickers; with it, I am instantly bolstered and prepared for whatever life throws at me. Like Calpol, cheese and red wine, I'll simply never not have it in the house.

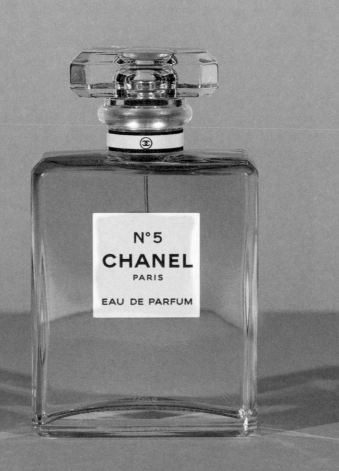

To choose a favourite red lipstick is impossible. You might as well ask me to name my favourite child. But ask me for the most iconic, and the answer comes easily. Ruby Woo is an ultra-bold phone-box red launched in 1999, effectively as a slightly more vivid, super-matte version of MAC's (already matte) Russian Red, the lipstick favoured by Madonna during the 'Who's That Girl?' and 'Blond Ambition' years (and consequently bought by me, of course). Ruby Woo became an instant bestseller and, until a Kardashian-Jenner told the world she wore its less interesting stablemate Velvet Teddy, was MAC's most popular lipstick – no mean feat when you have both a colour and formulation that's pretty hard for most women to wear. Ruby Woo is extremely matte. Glide silkily across the mouth like butter on hot toast, it does not. It more chugs along like wellies down a wet slide. What it gives in superb longevity, it robs in moisture. Its blue base, while fabulous for whitening teeth and making an impact, demands the level of confidence of a seasoned red-wearer.

But none of this matters, because Ruby Woo is meant to be a loud statement by an uncompromising woman. It's not meant to be pretty, it's designed to be fabulous, and on that it more than delivers. It looks glorious against extreme hair colours – platinum blonde or jet black – and on very pale, very olive or very dark skin (Dita Von Teese is a Ruby Woo fan – it looks sublime on her) and is the perfect vintage rockabilly red. It's the kind of lipstick that belongs with tattoos, leather jacket and a hoop petticoat, or maribou mules and mink stole. Since launching Ruby Woo, MAC has introduced a specially tweaked version for Ruby Woo fan Rihanna, called RiRi Woo, plus a much needed Ruby Woo liner, and a matching lip gloss. The latter rather misses the point for me. This is a true red shade for strong women who love proper lipstick, not for those who can't take the heat.

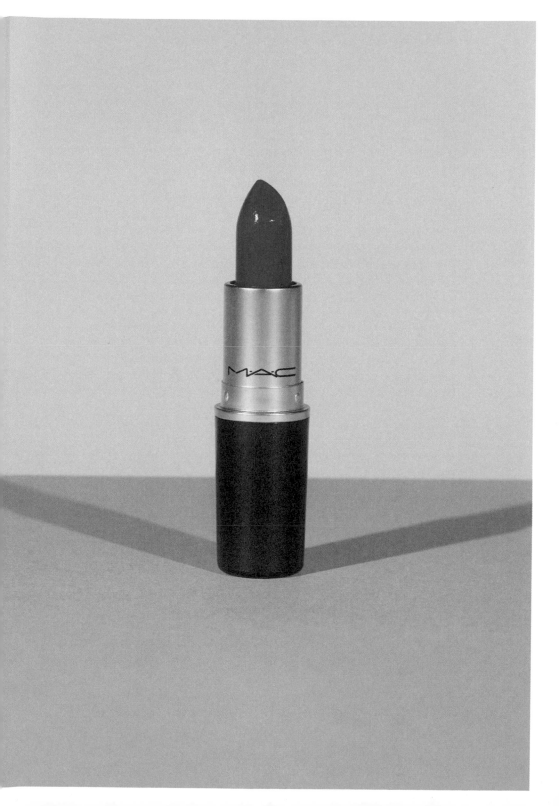

Similarly to boyfriends, I didn't realise how needlessly rubbish 99 per cent of hairdryers were – and still are – until I found a brilliant one. For years, I thought good haircuts existed only for one day, when a professional could magically dry them into shape. After that, I was on my own with the hot, noisy, smelly hunk of plastic that woke the kids, scared the dog and left my head with the functionality of a Van de Graaff generator. In Britain, they were bad. Plugged into an American hotel wall, they were tear-inducingly awful.

And then there was Parlux. These are professional dryers available in any salon supply store for the not inconsiderable sum of around £80/$120/100 euros. They're quite old-fashioned-looking (not in a particularly pretty way) and weigh about the same as a newborn baby in chainmail, which is why you should opt for the Compact model (already heavier than the average dryer) or the new Power Light, which have all the same features as their mother. All will style your hair in a way you previously thought impossible.

The impressively fast motor halves drying time, the three temperatures and speeds (in general, you want to start hot and fast and move down the settings during your blow dry, as a hairdresser would) give excellent shape and smoothness, and the high wattage makes a joke of your last dryer. Crucially, the Parlux has a proper cool shot setting, rather than a puny burst of tepid air offered by high street dryers. This allows you to properly set your style; leaving hair warm is like putting on a hot blouse straight from the ironing board. It'll ruin again in seconds. The unit is sturdy too. I've dropped my Parlux many times, and while I'd caution against recklessness, I must commend my 11-year-old dryer's stoicism – on and on it nobly goes. I've since moved on to a newer, similarly brilliant professional dryer (namely, the Hersheson) and bestowed the Parlux onto my gloriously thick-haired assistant, but only because the former is a little lighter. Age has not withered the Parlux, only weakened my right arm.

I find natural mascaras to be rather missing the point. I don't enhance my determinedly straight, short lashes to look like I have normal ones. I want them to be long, thick and fluttery like a Hereford cow's. I want good separation and a brush that coats hairs, not eyelids, and a formula that doesn't dry out in a matter of weeks. It seems so little to ask and yet is amazingly hard to find. It seems Pat McGrath, genius make-up artist, felt so similarly ill-served by the dramatic lash mascaras available that in 2001, she took a pile of toothbrushes backstage at the Dior catwalk show. The fat, dense bristles, when coated in black mascara, gave models a fanned, false lash effect that made lashes noticeable even to those sitting in the back row.

Inspired by McGrath's ingenuity, the product development team set about designing a commercially available mascara that created the same look as the somewhat impractical toothbrushes. The result was Diorshow, a sleek, elegant silver and black tube housing a fat brush that could perhaps clean the loo in a crisis. It was an instant bestseller and in my experience is the mascara most likely to make a red carpet appearance on a starlet's lashes. Make-up artists adore it, customers can't get enough of it. It gives lush, dark, bovine lashes to those previously deprived, layers brilliantly, and has good staying power on most. It smudges on me, but unless you're a serial mascara smudger, don't let that put you off – my dry skin is so thickly basted in greasy moisturiser that it could smudge a tattoo. Diorshow now comes in an additional, waterproof formula and several permanent and seasonal colours. Which is all very nice, but my mascara motto will always be Go Black or Go Home.

Sometimes a single beauty product is so huge, so instantly recognisable and ubiquitous, that it becomes an entire brand in its own right. Such is the case with this, the world's bestselling foundation and the base readers most often rave about at my events. Launched in 1997, Double Wear was designed to stay on, come what may, and it certainly does that. It doesn't transfer onto clothes and would probably survive nuclear holocaust to perfect the complexions of cockroaches and Keith Richards. Its shade range is ethnically inclusive, as is typical of American (as opposed to French) brands, its price is neither prohibitively obscene nor suspiciously low. The full coverage formula covers spots, blemishes, blotches, melasma and even faint scars but remains surprisingly comfortable to wear. It is, in my experience, what male and female popstars are most likely to wear on a hot, sweaty tour stage.

Despite my uneven skin pigmentation, Double Wear is not my own foundation of choice, because my skin is otherwise clear and to cover it so opaquely feels a little like throwing out the baby with the bathwater. Others criticise Double Wear's 'heavy' and not entirely natural-looking finish, but while I take their point (with the reminder that Double Wear still looks way more realistic than any foundation launched pre-1995), I'm not personally of the opinion that make-up's role should always be that of 'convincing liar' anyway. How joyless and dull. If that were the case, there'd be no red lipstick. An unthinkable tragedy indeed.

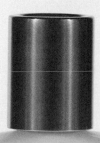

ESTĒE LAUDER

Double Wear
Stay-in-Place Makeup
Teint longue tenue
intransférable
SPF 10

In 1989 Clinique launched a new type of lip colour. Almost Lipstick was 'not quite a lipstick, not quite a gloss, but the best of both', and I was instantly intrigued. There were six shades in the range (Ruby Melt – the first sheer red I'd seen – was given to me by my brother David, much to my giddy joy), but the jewel in the crown was Black Honey, a blackberry stain without the jammy stickiness. Black Honey was so sheer, forgiving and thin of bullet (Almost Lipsticks came in a slender, stylo-type applicator) that it could be applied in mirrorless nightclub loos or standing on a bumpy night bus, or even while driving a car, as demonstrated by Julia Roberts, who slicks on Black Honey while behind the wheel in nineties film *Stepmom*. It made the wearer seem dressed up without looking try-hard. I was, and am, a huge fan myself and wore it throughout the nineties, but it looks good on literally everyone. As long as you had Black Honey in your kit, you could make any woman, regardless of age, race, hair or skin tone, look pretty great.

The rest of the shade line-up failed to make as much of an impact and so, some years later, Clinique axed Almost Lipsticks, leaving only bestseller Black Honey as a stand-alone product. I can think of few other examples of a single shade becoming so popular that it outlives its entire product line, but in this case it's wholly deserved. Clinique rolled again and relaunched Almost Lipsticks in the early 2000s, this time capitalising on its hero-shade's popularity by namechecking it throughout the rest of the range (Flirty Honey, Lovely Honey, Bare Honey and so on), but by now lip stains and tinted balms were ten a penny and the second-generation shades failed to take off. Almost Lipsticks were withdrawn yet again, with one inevitable exception. We're still sweet on Black Honey.

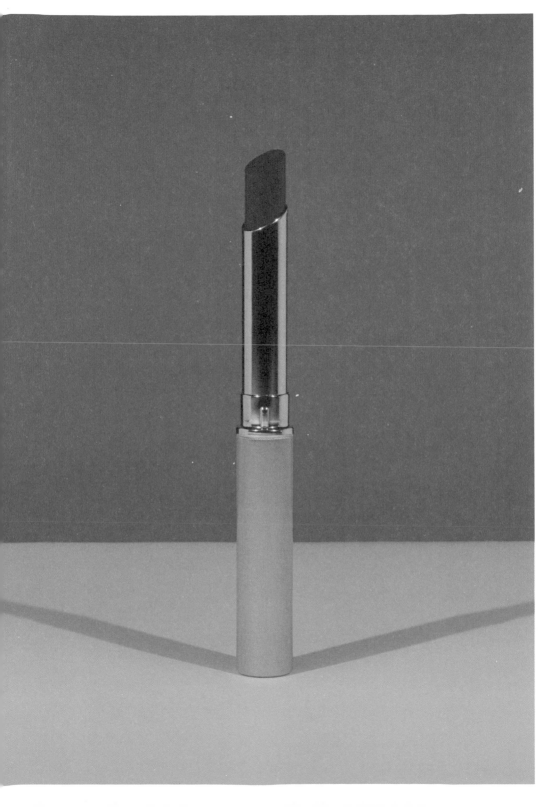

Max Factor's Creme Puff face powder is one of the first make-up items I was ever really aware of. As a tiny girl I would sit next to my grandmother on the bus and, as we neared our destination, watch her reach into her handbag for a gilt Stratton compact housing a pan of Creme Puff. She'd sweep the sponge over her nose and chin briskly and unfussily before clicking it shut, but just long enough for the strong, sweet baby powdery-smelling particles to become airborne and scent the whole top deck.

That Creme Puff smell, unchanged in six decades, still does strange things to me. It is one of the most instantly affecting, most nostalgic of fragrances. It smells of my nan, yes, but mostly Creme Puff just smells unapologetically of make-up (much like Dior lipstick does, or Bourjois powder rouge) at a time when make-up often smells of nothing at all. None of this sensitive skin molly-coddling, the Max Factor face powder hits you with a proper old-fashioned dressing-table smell and you'll bloody well like it. Fortunately, I love it. And if you've ever hovered over your gran's open handbag, trying to breathe in the interior's scent, then you will too.

Creme Puff is glamorous, feminine, special. It's not minimal, or pretending to be state of the art – it's an old-fashioned formula that made golden age Hollywood actresses like Ava Gardner, Vivien Leigh and Jean Harlow appear flawless and luminous on set. It continues to do the job extremely well today, in its seventh decade (though sadly, its nostalgia is misplaced in its Caucasian-only shade range). Creme Puff is soft and creamy, with excellent coverage, and gives a matte finish without ever looking chalky. It contains light-reflecting particles to mimic a smoother, clearer surface. It's perfect with retro red lips, black flicks and falsies, but also its full, layerable coverage makes it a great way to skip foundation on a more natural face – just brush over moisturiser and concealer. It's a product I use rarely, but I would never pack a full kit without it because sometimes it's exactly what a look needs, and the only thing that will do.

The Max Factor brand, founded by the man who literally invented the phrase 'make-up' (yes, really), is no longer sold in the States, where it first went on sale. I'd be very sad to see the same happen in Britain. We should cherish Creme Puff, beloved elder stateswoman of make-up and unarguably one of the most iconic beauty products of all time. I'm afraid it may be a case of use it now or lose it for ever.

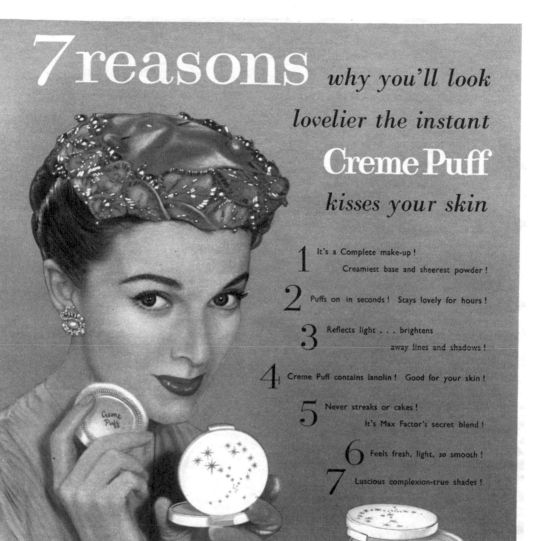

7 reasons

why you'll look

lovelier the instant

Creme Puff

kisses your skin

1 It's a Complete make-up!
   Creamiest base and sheerest powder!

2 Puffs on in seconds! Stays lovely for hours!

3 Reflects light . . . brightens
   away lines and shadows!

4 Creme Puff contains lanolin! Good for your skin!

5 Never streaks or cakes!
   It's Max Factor's secret blend!

6 Feels fresh, light, so smooth!

7 Luscious complexion-true shades!

The new complete make-up

Creme Puff *

by **MAX FACTOR** HOLLYWOOD . . . *the make-up that keeps its promise*

In Beautiful Mirror Compact with
luxury puff **7/9**
Refill, with luxury puff **4/11**
And a superb gilt compact, complete
with mirror and luxury puff **25/-**

My first foray into luxury skincare came via the Clarins catalogue, supposedly free but granted only after weeks of grooming a saleswoman who knew full well the schoolchild before her could barely afford a seven-inch single. I read this (and the 'Clinique Directory') like one might read a car repair manual, working out which products came in which order, where they were placed, how they might work, what they might do. The relative affordability of Clarins cleansing milks (and I really do mean relative, like gold to pavé-diamond platinum) made me save up my pocket money and Saturday job wages to get a bottle of my own, but not before I'd pinched some of my big brother's girlfriend's and sneakily refilled it with green Boots Natural Collection body lotion (I'm so sorry, Clare). It remains one of my more shameful decisions. I can only say in defence that I was stealing to invest in my future career.

Gratifyingly, the cleansers themselves (ivory 'With Gentian' and green 'With Alpine Herbs') remain unchanged since their launch in 1966 (the brand's first products after their plant oils and an absolutely extraordinary bust firming contraption that looks like an industrial funnel attached to a garden hose) and I applaud Clarins's apparent belief in 'if it ain't broke, don't fix it'. These cleansers really are still wonderful. They shift make-up very thoroughly when used with a hot cloth (though I tend to use them in the morning and a balm, cream or oil at night), they leave no sticky residue, only softness and comfort, and they smell blissfully cosying. The packaging has changed a little – I miss the fat, weighty glass bottles of my teenage dressing table – but the modern version maintains the simplicity of the old. The new squeezy cap does, however, prevent tampering, which in my case is probably for the best.

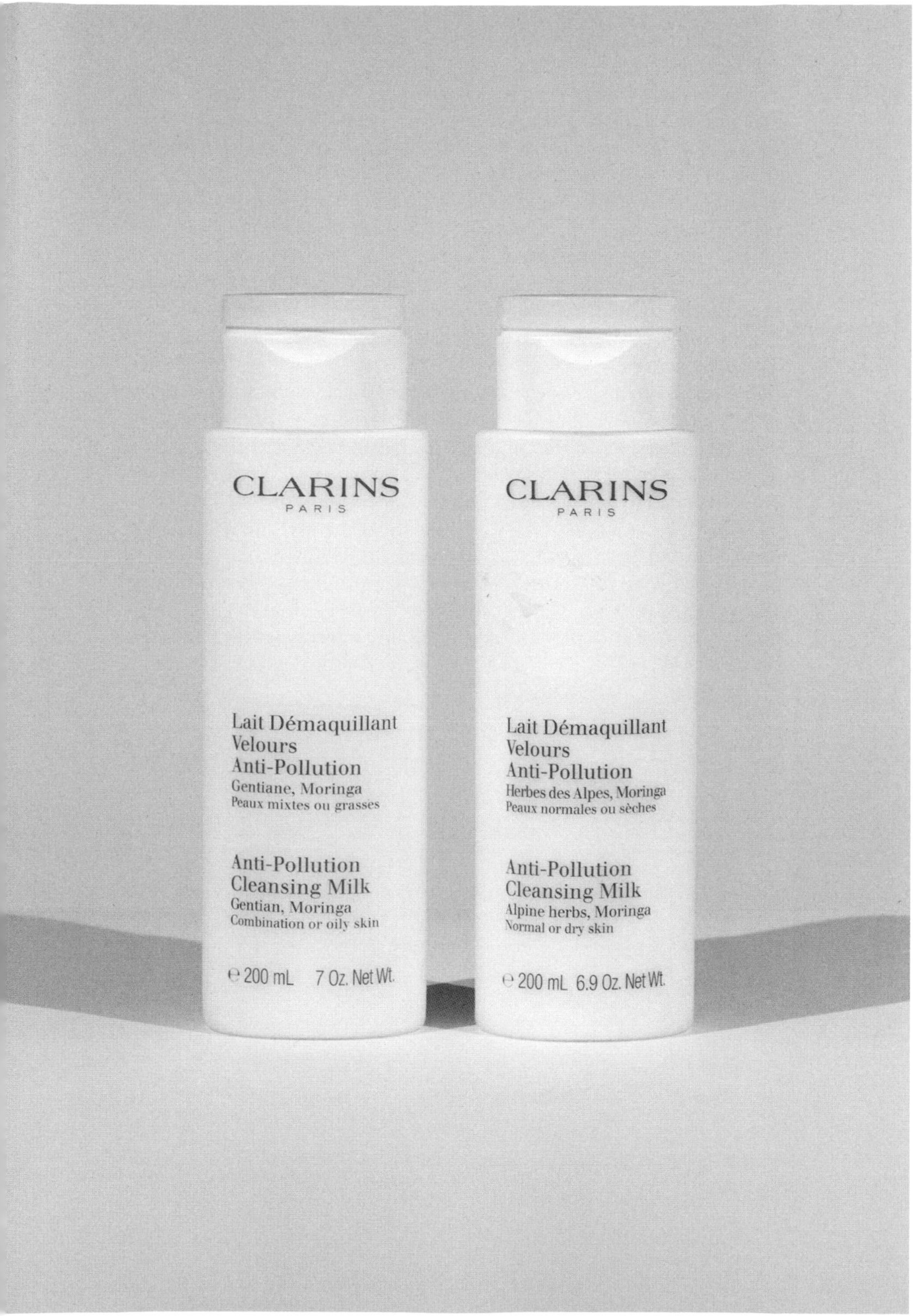
CLARINS
PARIS
Lait Démaquillant
Velours
Anti-Pollution
Gentiane, Moringa
Peaux mixtes ou grasses
Anti-Pollution
Cleansing Milk
Gentian, Moringa
Combination or oily skin
℮ 200 mL 7 Oz. Net Wt.
CLARINS
PARIS
Lait Démaquillant
Velours
Anti-Pollution
Herbes des Alpes, Moringa
Peaux normales ou sèches
Anti-Pollution
Cleansing Milk
Alpine herbs, Moringa
Normal or dry skin
℮ 200 mL 6.9 Oz. Net Wt.

When someone sits down to write the history of the nineties, they should do so in MAC Spice lip pencil. This reddy-brown liner became the Canadian-born professional brand's first 'hero product' and was *the* make-up accessory of the supermodel era; it graced a hundred glossy magazine covers and Linda Evangelista was never without it (I'm told she always conveniently needed to pee before shooting, then snuck on some Spice in the ladies' loo if the make-up artist had failed to). It became the look for a generation of girls like me, who thought it the height of sophistication to wear a lip pencil five shades darker than the lips it outlined. After making a pilgrimage to buy my first Spice in Harvey Nichols (MAC's only UK stockist at that time), and having nicked my mum's peach CoverGirl lipstick, I debuted the look at a Salt-N-Pepa concert in Newport leisure centre. The band failed to show up but I didn't care because I felt a million dollars.

Spice subsequently accompanied me to acid house clubs, to gigs and on capers, out on dates with inappropriate men. It accessorised Kookai hotpants, Lycra frocks from Pineapple, smiley T-shirts and red Kickers. I teamed it with fishnets, a velvet choker and beret and imagined myself in an Ellen von Unwerth shoot. I wore it with jeans and a wide headband and felt like Bardot, with a football shirt and Adidas Gazelles and thought I was Christy Turlington on the John Galliano catwalk. I was far from any of these things, but look back on Spice without a moment's regret because, unlike so many products that completely sum up a fleeting moment in life, Spice is still a much loved, often used, part of my beauty kit. Only nowadays I wear Spice with a matching lipstick of brick red or terracotta brown, not a contrasting gloss the colour of Elastoplast.

The age of the selfie has reintroduced so many old-fashioned beauty techniques that I'd quite happily have left in the history books with lead face powder and chastity belts, and yet I feel nothing but joy at the huge resurgence in popularity of false eyelashes. Falsies were invented in 1916 (later than one might perhaps imagine), on the set of the film *Intolerance*, for leading actress Seena Owen's big close-up. The director wanted the lashes on Owen's sad eyes to skim her cheeks, and so the film's hairdresser threaded wig hair onto some gauze and glued it to her lashline. Reusable false lashes went into production – initially using real hair or animal fur – and became a key element in almost all iconic Hollywood beauty looks. Nowadays, lashes are synthetic and mainly come on strips, but there's still something so brilliantly decadent and utterly mad about sticking fake hair onto eyelids with glue, something so satisfying about fluttering huge lashes more at home on Tweetie Pie. No one can be bothered every day, of course, but the occasional application of falsies is a wonderful thing when you know how – and it really is so much easier than you may fear.

First, the lashes must be cut to size (unless they're half lashes – those designed to be worn on the outer corners only and often just the thing for a more natural look). Cutting is important because if a strip lash is even the tiniest bit too wide for your lids, then the end will hit the bridge of your nose and peel off at some point during the course of the night, and a droopy falsie is never a good look. Cut from the outside; it's tempting to preserve maximum flutter and cut from the inside, but this will rob the fan-shape of its gradual incline, and look unnatural. Second, always, always allow the glue (preferably Duo) to become a little dry and tacky. Wet glue is too messy and makes the lash too mobile and prone to wandering maddeningly onto fingers during application. Third, apply a little black liner and black mascara to disguise any joins. That's it.

There are hundreds of wonderful lashes on the market. I love MAC 20, Red Cherry Joan, We Are Faux Carey Red and a host of designs by Eylure, but the affordable drugstore brand Ardell makes my favourites of all – and not only because of their deliciously naff 1970s branding. Ardell's selection of designs is vast and caters for all eye sizes and tastes: from spiky and Twiggy-like to sleepy noir-era Bacall, to sumptuous feline flutters à la Loren. They either come without glue (my preference) or with Duo (the best). The invisible bands mean they can be worn more convincingly by chemotherapy patients than many other lashes, and, on a similarly practical level, they come out of the packaging without tearing or warping, go on like a dream and the tapered shapes and soft materials ensure that, generally speaking, they look more Old Hollywood, less Spearmint Rhino.

Among my earliest memories is one of lying on a towel as a young toddler, fresh from the bath, toasty from the nearby coal fire, giggling hysterically as my grandmother 'iced me like a birthday cake' with Johnson's Baby Lotion, squeezed direct from the bottle like a piping bag. Forty years on, it remains one of my favourite smells of all time. It's the smell of comfort, of security, of uncomplicated and predictable times. One deep whiff is like being cosseted in a warm blanket and tucked tightly and cosily into a single bed. It's a fragrance I always think of as smelling exactly how it looks – pink, mellow, delicate, old-fashioned, soft and sweet. It's frankly no good on my dry skin (it works as a cleanser for light make-up at a push, and is a nice body lotion for normal skins), but I love the smell so much that I'm never without a bottle in the house. If I feel inexplicably sad or stressed out, I flip open the cap and inhale.

I feel about Beauty Flash the way I feel about olives: I should like them, they're very much my kind of thing, other people love them and I doggedly keep trying to join in, but I just can't pull it off. This is a balm that goes over moisturiser to plump and blur lines, pep up tiredness and general haggishness, but on me – and apparently me alone – it has always peeled off in clumps as soon as I attempt to apply make-up over the top. No matter, because what is indisputable is Beauty Flash's iconic status. This is the product, I think, that first tabled the notion of primer – a skincare/make-up hybrid to smooth and perfect the complexion in readiness for foundation. There was nothing else like it when I first tried it some twenty-six years ago, and while things may have since moved on considerably to include primers for every conceivable skin type and gripe, blur balms and light reflectors for instant de-ageing, and so on, Beauty Flash's countless fans remain utterly devoted to the original. I almost envy them.

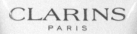

**Baume
Beauté Eclair**
Eclaire le visage,
retend les traits

**Beauty Flash
Balm**
Brightens, tightens

If beauty had a grande dame, an impossibly glamorous French nana, who turned up at parties in a great dress and smoked Sobranie cigarettes through a Bakelite holder, she would be Guerlain's Météorites. These are multicoloured pastel pearls of face powder designed to be swirled together with a brush then buffed into the skin to brighten and illuminate. Launched in 1987, Météorites may have looked outwardly like an antique shop find, but was remarkably ahead of its time. For years, it was one of very few consumer powders designed to give the complexion a radiant, rather than matte, finish (the radiance trend didn't really hit the mainstream until Revlon launched Skinlights over a decade later), and the first to introduce the concept of powder balls (or 'pearls'), allowing several different colours or shades to be used simultaneously to give a multi-dimensional look, before technology could provide it in traditional pressed formulations. Météorites was prohibitively expensive for many, but hugely influential on the mass market. Body Shop, Boots and Avon soon made bronzer, blusher and face powder in pearls, taking them from inaccessible luxury to full-on beauty craze. Météorites remained aloof and became a beauty icon with a devoted cult following.

Nowadays, illuminating powders are ten a penny and I won't pretend that Météorites is my own weapon of choice, but I'm not sure I'd have so many to choose from were it not for Guerlain's trailblazing. The pearls come in a stained-panel pot not a million miles from a Tiffany lamp, which when opened, releases the delicious powdery fug of crushed Parma Violet sweets. The whole thing is bulky, breakable and wholly impractical for any manner of travel, and should be moored to some art nouveau dressing table next to a string of beads and a Dirty Martini. But Guerlain has made some concessions to modernity: there are now different colourways for more skin tones, pressed versions, travel containers and various seasonal limited editions. Each is as unfeasibly pretty as the next.

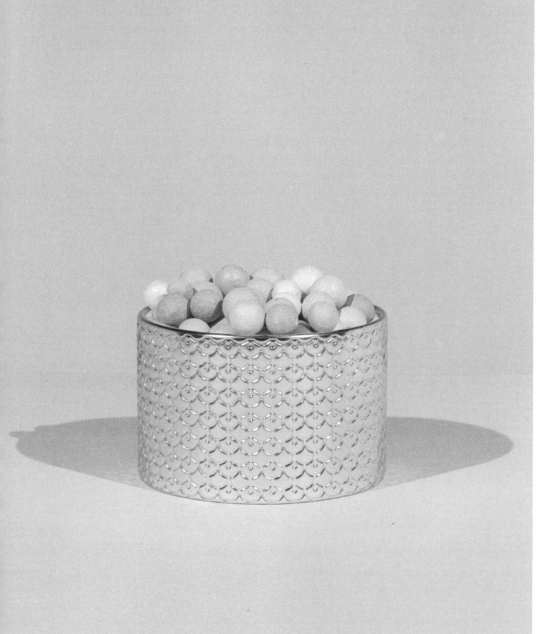

There was a time in the late eighties/early nineties when a 79-cent pot of Carmex lip balm had as much cachet as an army surplus-store MA1 flight jacket and selvedge Levi's – perhaps more, since it had to be scored in an American drugstore and flown home. The opaque glass jar topped with a bright yellow printed tin cap, almost entirely unchanged since its 1937 launch by cold-sore sufferer Alfred Woelbing, represented the kind of vintage Americana we Brits were already lapping up via Levi's 501 commercials, Dax Wax and Athena airbrush prints of James Dean.

But those in the industry were ostensibly more concerned with its contents. Unlike Vaseline and Blistex, Carmex had a matte finish. It didn't interfere with the shine-free lipsticks of the day, and didn't cause lip pencils to lose friction and veer off-course. It was utilitarian, serious, slightly butch. All budding and actual make-up artists carried it in their kit and for many years the staple make-up look for all male models and musicians on shoots was 'foundation, Kryolan concealer, powder, Guerlain bronzer, clear mascara, Carmex' (I couldn't tell you how many times I dutifully performed this routine). Off set and away from the industry, there was great snob-value in pulling a jar of Carmex from your mini backpack and so understandably, but somewhat disappointingly, Carmex saw their chance and soon the balm was available in UK pro-supply stores and fashion boutiques (including the original Space NK, which also sold juices, handbags and frocks) and later even Boots and Superdrug. It led the way for Smith's Rosebud Salve – another nostalgically tin-packaged balm – and for Vaseline to repackage its petroleum jelly in a flat tin and rebrand it as 'Lip Therapy'.

With the curse of accessibility and the benefit of perspective, Carmex lost its allure. Its shine-free finish is still useful, if no longer unique, but its lip-saving capabilities are bettered elsewhere. I find men still love the camphor smell, non-greasy feel and ungirlie packaging, which occasionally gets a limited edition makeover (the recent Peanuts/Snoopy and superheroes collaborations were a well-conceived delight). I rarely use it now, but always keep a pot in my kit to remind me of exciting times and endless possibilities, and for the occasional mentholated whiff of an industry that was to change my life for ever.

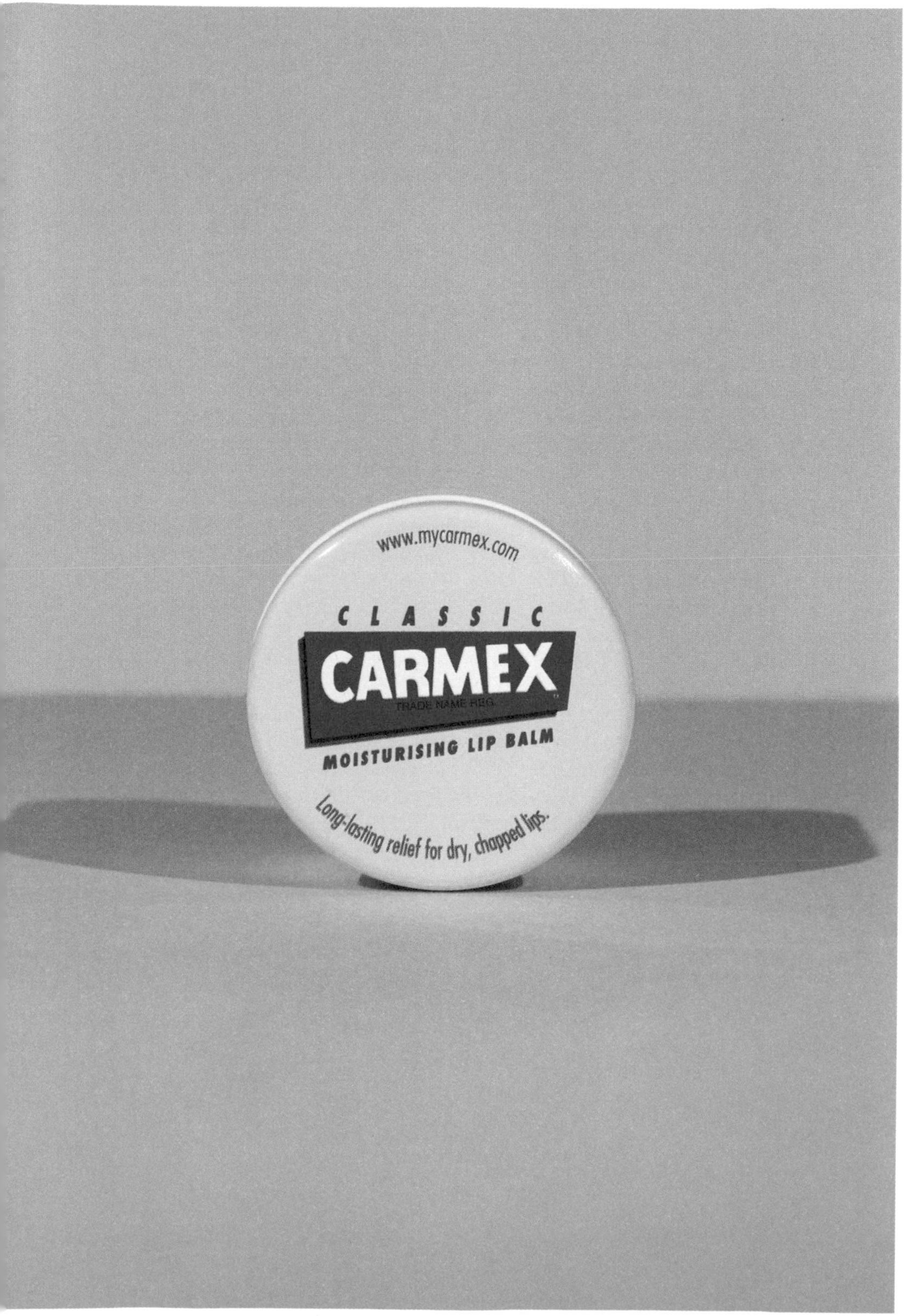
www.mycarmex.com
CLASSIC
CARMEX
TRADE NAME REG.
MOISTURISING LIP BALM
Long-lasting relief for dry, chapped lips.

One can almost chart British society's increasing liberality through the growing confidence with which the average woman asks a Nars sales assistant for an Orgasm. As recently as 2010, the inclusion of this powder blusher in my *Guardian Weekend* beauty column prompted one reader to accuse me of wilfully setting up the women of Britain for humiliation. All I could say is that it's worth a moment's shame, because Nars Orgasm is a must. I can think of few other colour cosmetics – least of all, complexion products – that genuinely look pretty on every skin tone, from white to olive to brown to black. The clue is in the name. This is a blusher designed to mimic the flush of colour to the cheeks at sexual climax or, in less florid language, it makes you look just-shagged. A smart and attention-grabbing way to market a product, for sure. Orgasm launched in 1999 and its name certainly helped it get plenty of publicity and celebrity endorsement (Jennifer Lopez, at the height of her fame, was rarely seen without it), but it's still absolutely true that just like a climactic rush of blood to the face, Nars Orgasm makes almost everyone look better.

The secret is Orgasm's perfectly balanced mix of peach and pink pigments that both brightens pale or sallow complexions and neutralises rosy ones, and teams with red and pink lipstick as well as it matches apricots and peach. A subtle, shimmery gold fleck stops it ever looking ashy or chalky on dark skins. This universal quality is what makes Orgasm not only Nars's biggest seller (120 are sold every hour of the day), but also the matriarch of an entire franchise including spin-offs like Super Orgasm (a hyper-glittery version of the original), the Multiple Orgasm (a stick creme blush and an open goal for the product namers, let's face it), a nail polish, lip gloss and illuminator. But none is as indispensable as the original. I'd only discourage its use on those whose cheeks are scarred or bumpy, as Orgasm's slight shimmer will do them no favours. But I'd urge those same women to simply choose another (ideally matte) shade from Nars's range, perhaps Sex Appeal or Zen. Because while it's impossible to describe any brand as the best at everything, I have no hesitation in declaring Nars the very best at blush.

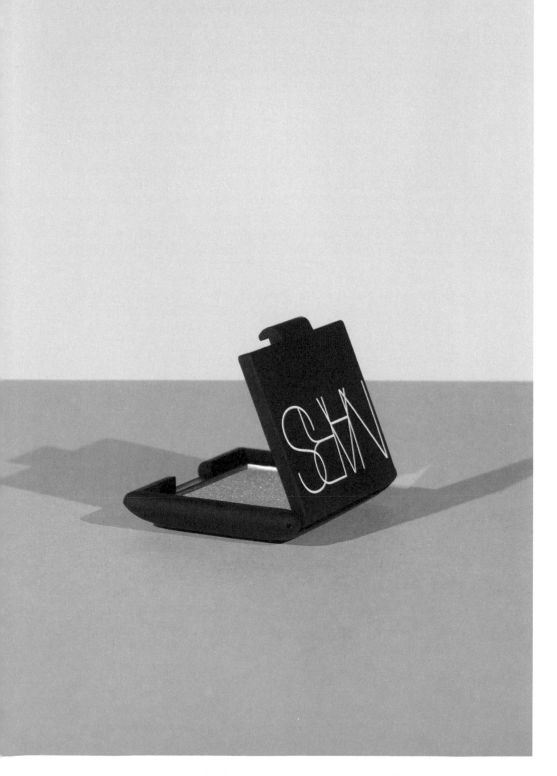

Clinique is my first love, and alongside a hereditary skin condition that saw me in and out of dermatologists' offices throughout my childhood, sparked my enduring passion for skincare. Like every woman I know, I still have many of Clinique's products on my bathroom shelf and dressing table (you will need to prise Bottom Lash Mascara, Take The Day Off Cleansing Oil and Superbalm from my cold dead hands), and yet I haven't used its iconic and revolutionary 3-Step skincare system for decades. But I still give it huge credit and reverence, because much like a teenage boyfriend who introduced me to great music and nightlife, but ultimately wasn't for me, 3-Step represents a moment of awakening and explosion in my curiosity and knowledge.

The three-part regime, developed by respected dermatologist Dr Norman Orentreich and Estée Lauder executive Carol Phillips in 1968 (and barely changed since, the addition of a little hydrating hyaluronic acid aside), comprises a facial soap, four numbered salicylic acid liquid exfoliators of increasing strength (at time of writing, a new alcohol-free version is in the pipeline), and a pale yellow moisturiser for all skin types. Fragrance-free and allergy tested – unheard of in those days – it introduced the concept of exfoliation (the removal of dead skin cells to reveal brighter, newer, smoother skin beneath) to the masses, was the first nationally available dermatologist's range (others were sold locally, in anonymous medication bottles direct from doctors' offices), and, as such, revolutionised the entire cosmetics industry. Customers were given an on-counter analysis using a 'computer' (and when I say computer, I mean something that nowadays has more in common with an abacus), and prescribed the specific soap and clarifying lotion for their needs.

In 3-Step, Clinique also introduced the concept of functional, rather than needlessly fancy, premium skincare for the masses, and its packaging – pared down, clean, stylish and minimal – was photographed by the great still life photographer Irving Penn in a series of iconic advertisements without model or figurehead, cleverly appealing to all women, regardless of age, colour or skin type. The products, dressed only with a toothbrush, were sold as the new basics: the white T-shirt and jeans of every woman's skincare wardrobe, onto which all other lotions or potions were to be layered. This core message – three simple products and three quick steps for better skin – proved enormously successful and endures to this day, and provided the basis for an entire brand of simple, effective, problem-solving cosmetics upon which so many of us still rely.

And yet despite the fact that it remains the world's bestselling skincare routine, 3-Step can still be described as a cult. Women (and men – the Clinique For Men range differs only in packaging) who love 3-Step, *really* love it, and will countenance no other regime. And I certainly won't argue – I've seen tremendous results on skin of all ages. Personally, I simply cannot get on board with facial soap in any guise; there are liquid exfoliants I prefer (though they might not exist if it weren't for Clinique's groundbreaking Clarifying Lotion), and the mighty Dramatically Different Moisturizing Lotion isn't mighty enough for my naturally drier-than-sawdust face. But none of this matters. It works for millions, it may work for you, and no one can begin to deny that it permanently changed how most of us see skincare. Clinique 3-Step changed the world, and respect is very much due.

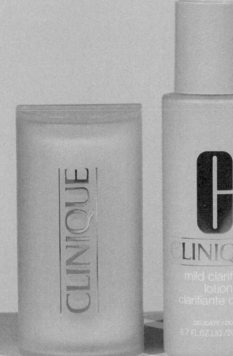
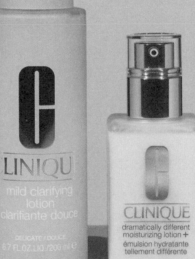

I can never lay claim to being a great lover of natural skincare. Ethics are certainly important, and I am all for paraben-free if that's important to you (the evidence against them is woolly at best, and most of us eat parabens every day, so I'm sceptical, to say the least). I'm certainly a lover of many essential oils and balm cleansers, I choose organic milk to pour in my tea, boil organic eggs for my breakfast, but when it comes to skincare, my priorities are efficacy and results – and in my view, those usually come from a combination of the best of both science and nature, not from homeopathy for its own sake.

Skin Food, by Swiss-German health shop beauty brand Weleda, is a notable exception. It's a rich, unctuous and affordable balm made from 100 per cent natural ingredients like almond oil, beeswax, calendula, rosemary, pansy and chamomile, for the purpose of moisturising dry faces and bodies. There's something so lovely about its slightly medicinal metal tube and 1970s earth mother green design. But the product, sold at a rate of one every thirty seconds, is the real star here. Used by Victoria Beckham, Alexa Chung, Julia Roberts, Winona Ryder, Adele, a million models, make-up artists and, erm, me to baste my face like a turkey on long-haul flights, Skin Food acts as the name suggests: it's exactly what to reach for when your skin feels peckish for something lovely, and leaves face and body snug, cosseted and comfy. I adore its gorgeous botanical smell, its reasonable price point, its assured place next to mung beans and nut bars in health food stores, its integrity and modesty. But most of all, I love that Skin Food has steadfastly stuck to its guns through every imaginable beauty trend and, almost a hundred advertising-free years after launching, is as relevant and more widely loved than ever, like some kindly great-grandmother who always quietly knew best.

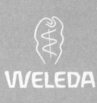

WELEDA

Skin Food

for dry
and rough skin

Skin Food

Touche Éclat is arguably the most iconic make-up item of all time. The evidence can be seen everywhere: make-up artists referring to a 'touche éclat look' (as one might use the term 'Hoover' for vacuum cleaner) when they actually just mean the artificial adding of brightness; men raiding their wives' make-up bags for an instant pick-me-up; women who own no other make-up keeping a regular stock to perk up sleepless eyes; a thousand copycat products; sales figures so vast that this one gold tube is a brand all on its own. But oh, Touche Éclat, our own relationship is complicated. I first discovered this elegant gold clicky pen of salmon-pink cream in the early nineties, when it had secured its place in every make-up artist's kit I invariably poked my nose into. The buzz escalated outside the professional world, partly thanks to the explosion of celebrity culture and countless 'What's in my make-up bag' interviews with A–Z list actresses and popstars, all wildly singing its praises. Somewhere in this process, Touche Éclat became known as a concealer, and this, for me, is where my issues began.

Touche Éclat is not a concealer. It is a brightening corrector, and one launched way before any other mainstream brands had considered their usefulness (nowadays, correctors are everywhere). On white skin, its sheer pinky hue helps cancel out grey tones commonly found under the eyes, and highlights cheekbones to make them pop. It does not cover spots, blemishes, patches of sun damage or much else for that matter, and to misappropriate it is often to make things much worse. When flicking through a wedding photo album on Facebook, I can invariably spot Touche Éclat before I've even had time to digest the frock. When worn in abundance as a generic cover-all, with no proper concealer over the top, it creates the impression of a fortnight spent skiing in goggles in Val d'Isère. On dark skins, the original shade (called Radiant Touch, it has now rightly been joined by several brand extensions, including more skin tones, colour correctors for different uses, and a very good light-reflecting foundation) looked sickly and unnatural.

Its woeful misuse was and is a terrible shame, because when used judiciously and sparingly as an undercoat for concealer or as a straightforward highlighter, Touche Éclat is actually rather wonderful. Its revolutionary click pen packaging makes it very convenient for making up on the move (you'll need to wash the brush regularly, of course), its thin formula blends beautifully, and its sparkle-free light reflection is perfect on brow bones to sharpen their appearance. On cheekbones, or applied lightly across the centre of the face in a cat's whiskers formation (then blended, of course), it can bathe skin in gloriously flattering light.

Sadly, my appreciation for Touche Éclat came way too late in the day. I am horribly allergic (and I say this as someone who, after a lifetime of product testing, has skin as hardy as Shane MacGowan's liver), and so I cannot finally make amends for my former harshness. I use Bobbi Brown or Becca corrector on my own dark circles. But to the vast majority of women who can click, sweep and blend Touche Éclat with no adverse effects, all I can say is that I finally see where you're coming from.

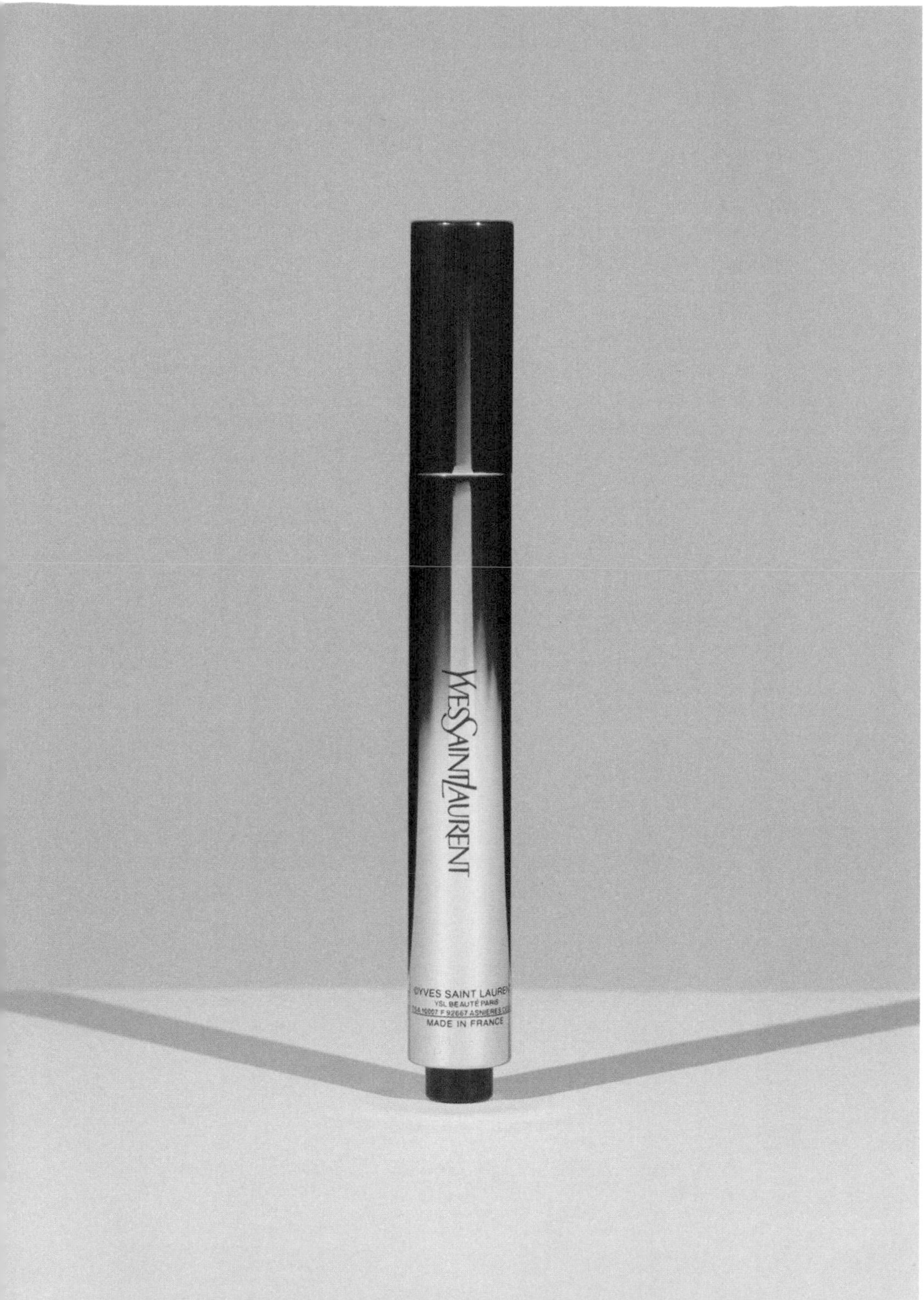
YVES SAINT LAURENT
YSL BEAUTÉ PARIS
MADE IN FRANCE

I do so love a product with a sneaky sideline in something for which it was never designed. KY Jelly as a hair styler on short retro haircuts, non-oily eye make-up remover on stubborn carpet and soft furnishing stains, and clear nail polish on freshly laddered tights are just a few hugely satisfying deployments of products entirely fit for multiple purpose. Perhaps the most polymathic product of all is this, a cheap-as-chips fragrant body moisturising spray, reportedly used for decades by the US Navy as a standard-issue mosquito spray for soldiers stationed abroad. Meanwhile, on Civvy Street, Skin So Soft's vast legion of fans (40 million bottles have been sold since its 1961 launch, and Avon representatives stockpile it at the beginning of every summer) claim the dry-oil spray makes an excellent remover for candlewax, chewing gum and paint. Artists and decorators use it to clean brushes, housekeepers swear by it to remove carpet stains, and Hollywood film crews douse themselves in large quantities before entering an insect-ridden shooting location. Even the royal household is rumoured to use it for purposes on which we can only speculate.

What we can be sure of is that Skin So Soft is a hidden gem of a product, and that to have this somewhat dated and naff-looking bottle (more like something kept under the sink than in the bathroom cabinet) handy at all times is to be in on an immensely satisfying secret. So wide is Skin So Soft's skill set that it's easy to forget that it delivers admirably on its original brief. It has a light, pleasant smell, a non-greasy texture, and leaves limbs softened and more evenly toned. And mercifully abhorrent to mozzies.

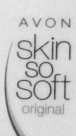

AVON

skin
so
soft

original

dry oil spray

huile sèche en
vaporisateur

+ jojoba

150 ml ℮

I admire beauty brands with a sort of benign arrogance about their star products, a self-belief so strong that to tweak, reformulate or move with the times would be an unthinkable admission that any improvement on the original is even possible. This is why I so admire Elizabeth Arden's Eight Hour Cream, a thick, glossy, greasy preparation invented in the 1930s by Miss Arden herself and used ever since on the burns, cuts, windburn, chapping, grazes, dry lips, ragged cuticles and unruly brows of humans, and on the aching legs of thoroughbred horses (yes, really – Miss Arden always kept jars in her stable and it caught on. I suppose if you're dropping half a million on an animal, then twenty quid on some luxury hoof ointment is mere loose change).

But modern beauty fans will know 8-Hour less as a medicinal balm, more as a multi-purpose gloss quite unlike the rest. While other paraffin-based products like Vaseline become thin and slide gradually off the skin or into the eyes, 8-Hour remains thick, holds its gel-like structure well and tends to stay firmly (and stickily) on the job. This makes it peerless in changing the consistency and finish of all manner of traditional cosmetics. Make-up artists mix it with powder shadows to create eye gloss, with kohl to make brow wax, with lipstick for a sheer lip gloss or gleaming flush of cheek colour. But this is no industry secret. It's by far Elizabeth Arden's most successful product, with a tube of the original formula (as opposed to its many spin-offs) selling every thirty seconds worldwide. Millions of women, including Victoria Beckham, Penélope Cruz, Emma Watson and Kate Moss, use 8-Hour neat to add a flattering sheen to cheekbones and lips, softening the skin and adding a very subtle pinky-peach tint. I see 8-Hour primarily as cosmetic, but I don't quibble with its skincare benefits in certain applications – the mild beta hydroxy acids slough dead skin flakes, particularly on the mouth and nose – while the vitamin E and paraffin provide temporary moisture and relief.

Those who love 8-Hour seem never to be without a tube in their handbag, ready for emergency deployment, and will suggest its use in seemingly any skin crisis or extreme weather condition. It provides an almost unmovable barrier of emollient and for this reason, many women even swear by 8-Hour for basting the face in readiness for long-haul flights, though some of us really wish they wouldn't; the smell is a pungent and not universally pleasing combination of roses, lanolin, a nana's handbag and Germolene. The relatively new unscented version – though by no means odourless – is a tad more sociable, if a little inauthentic.

To the young or disinterested, bath bombs must have just appeared from nowhere, piled high in Lush shop windows, their distinctive and sometimes obnoxious smell polluting the air for fifty yards. But for me, bath bombs will always be a reminder of Cosmetics-to-Go, Lush's innovative forerunner in Poole, Dorset. This was the first incarnation of Lush, founded in 1987 by husband and wife Mo and Mark Constantine and beauty therapist Liz Weir, selling natural, British-made and faintly bonkers products like solid shampoo bars, fresh fruit-enzyme face masks hand blended on the premises like smoothies, peanut butter face scrubs that were literally good enough to eat, and Second World War-inspired liquid stockings in glass bottles that looked like Camp Coffee. Like the Body Shop's errant, less neurotic little sister (the Constantines had invented many products for Anita Roddick's fledgling empire, including its bestselling Cocoa Butter Hand & Body Lotion), Cosmetics-to-Go was the first time I'd seen beauty with both a sense of humour and a strong sense of purpose.

A cruelty-free stance was at the heart of the brand, without it becoming so worthy and earnest as to be dull. Quite the contrary: I looked forward to new Cosmetics-to-Go catalogues like new issues of *Just Seventeen*, and pored over the quirky illustrations and chatty copy. I'd then ring the order line whenever I had a spare couple of quid, and two days later, a brown paper-wrapped box covered in primary-coloured labels would arrive, crammed with truly groundbreaking and extraordinarily packaged products. Eyeshadows in faux-marble wedges, popped in a Camembert box to create a bespoke palette not a million miles from a Trivial Pursuit wheel, a men's grooming range festooned in chintzy florals when everyone else was flogging aftershaves got up to look like car parts, and a blackberry-scented bath powder moulded to look like the kind of Acme bomb beloved of Wile E. Coyote. This was the first 'bath bomb' – a fizzing mix of fragrance, essential oils, moisturising butters, citric acid and bicarbonate of soda, directly inspired by the uplifting, soothing qualities of Alka-Seltzer. Its relative cheapness and versatility spawned a whole range of bombs in multiple shapes, colours and scents, and an entirely new product category was born.

Ultimately, Cosmetics-to-Go had too many brilliant and impractical ideas, too little business acumen. Even as a child, I wondered how they could possibly be making enough money when, as a matter of course, they'd mistakenly send me free duplicates of practically every order I placed. They weren't, as it turned out. Cosmetics-to-Go went down the plughole in 1994, but their bath bombs stayed afloat, providing the old CTG team with a basis for new venture Lush, now a hugely successful British high street retailer based on the same environment/employee/animal-friendly principles as before. Lush still makes dozens of different bath bombs (selling well over 26 million of them to date), all copied endlessly by rivals, often with much less care for quality and ethics. Even when the real thing enters my house via press sample, kid's birthday gift or party bag, my heart sinks in anticipation of post-bath scrubbing to remove some glittery lurid puce tidemark. But I always give in to the pleas and chuck one in because I want my kids to see that modern beauty products aren't only for making someone's nose look skinny on Instagram. They can also be fun, kitsch, bonkers and kind. No one demonstrates that better than Lush. Long may they fizz.

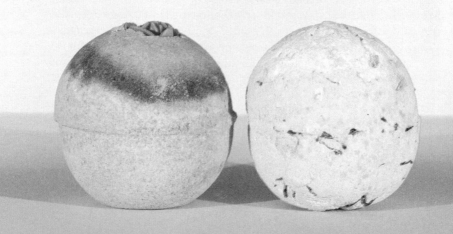

Any company awarded a Royal Warrant – a recognition of excellence for selected small firms that supply the royal households – must be doing something right. A firm granted Royal Warrants by nine successive sovereigns, though, can claim quite persuasively to be doing pretty much everything better than anyone else. Founded in 1777, the brush-making concern G.B. Kent & Sons was awarded its first warrant by George III and has received royal thumbs-up from every king and queen since. Kent, the UK's longest established brush-maker, is a heart-swelling example of a firm peopled by artisans, preserving specialist skills in the face of mass production and foreign imports.

Kent allies British pluck and ingenuity – the Second World War saw the firm produce a shaving brush with a secret compartment for map and compass to facilitate the escape of prisoners of war – with meticulous production methods to produce doughty, tactile artefacts of enduring loveliness. Its saw-cut combs are polished and buffed by hand, the teeth free of the tiny, snaggy ridges found in injection-moulded combs. The women's tail comb – a seventies classic that sells a pleasingly un-mass-market forty a day – is a sleek, frictionless delight that makes you want to keep on combing, mermaid-like, long after the practical necessity has gone. I like to imagine Princess Anne using one to tease her crown before sweeping everything into a no-nonsense riding bun, or Charles reaching for his Kent brush in the hope of making his remaining strands go further.

If sharing a brush supplier with the Queen doesn't float your royal yacht – and I do understand – focus instead on the preciousness of British-made beauty tools, made with love, pride and devotion to the craft, and sold widely at a very reasonable and accessible price point (my paternal grandfather always carried a tortoiseshell Kent – and he was a lowly stable lad). Kent is a company I wish to exist for ever. We should never assume that's a given, and perhaps replace our old combs forthwith.

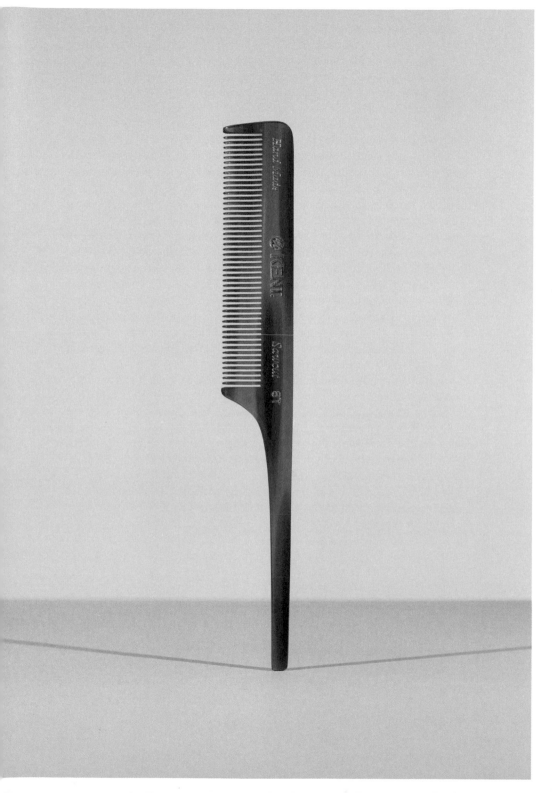

In the eyes of critics, perhaps no product better sums up the madness of beauty than the eyelash curler. Here is a prohibitively dangerous-looking piece of metal that resembles something a Victorian dentist might use to winch out a rotting molar, used for the sole purpose of lifting and curving one's eyelashes temporarily. It does seem slightly bonkers, on reflection. And yet, with the right curler, it really is a uniquely gratifying twenty-second job.

The Shu Uemura eyelash curler is such a reference point for all other beauty tools, that it's easy to forget that it only launched in 1991. When Japanese make-up artist Shu Uemura launched his groundbreaking eponymous brand, there were few luxury lash curlers on the market and he felt all of them failed to sufficiently and comfortably curl short lashes. And so he briefed his son Hiroshi Uemura to create one that did. Hiroshi worked with professional make-up artists to test different widths, lengths, gradient curves, rubber elasticity and pressure intensity until he had what the professionals still believe to be the eyelash curler against which all others should be measured. And while to the untrained eye it may look the same as a three quid version in Boots, they are apples and oranges. The Shu Uemuras don't pinch or bend lashes in an unflattering right angle. They can be used both under and over mascara (this is always my preference – you get a better hold) without damage and even on short, pin-straight lashes like mine they give great and lasting curve. The mechanism is loose enough to allow partial release of tension, but can be tightened in case it becomes slack.

At time of writing, Shu Uemura's eyelash curler has won a major beauty award for fifteen consecutive years and in all that time I don't think I've met a single make-up artist who doesn't own at least one set. The curler has appeared on magazine covers (Kylie Minogue's iconic 1991 shoot for *The Face*), in films (*The Devil Wears Prada*, where it's namechecked) and in pop videos (Annie Lennox's wonderful 'Why' promo, featuring the extraordinary make-up skills of the great Martin Pretorius – a must-see for any beauty nerd), and been honoured with several limited editions, including a twenty-four-carat gold version. Shu Uemura's eyelash curler is a beauty icon because, quite simply, it's the best.

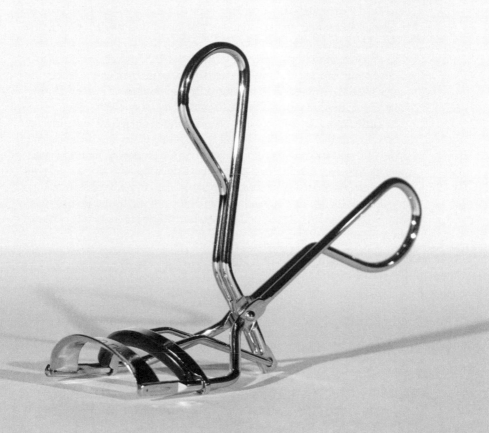

There are few products more cheering than a little fat pot of Bourjois blush or eyeshadow, nor as instantly recognisable. None of us has lived in a time where these multicoloured pastel powders didn't line high street chemist racks like freshly baked macarons in a patisserie window. These are domed, single shadows and blushers in sheer, muted tones including matriarch Cendre de Rose, an old Hollywood rouge, the deep, black-red hue of crushed rose petals, released in 1881, and Rose Thé, a dusky nude-pink blush born in 1936. For over 150 years, these traditional powders have provided the basis for the entire Bourjois brand, however cutting edge the rest of its offering has become.

The Fard Pastel powders – now known as Pastel Joues – are baked (much like Chanel's European market shadows; for years, rumours abounded that they were made in the same factory) and so colour payoff is not as dramatic as with a modern, pressed pigment powder, but the finish is soft and blendable, and the colours are gentle, pretty washes that are hard to get wrong. Their rose scent is blissful, reminiscent of the dusty, flowery interior of a great-granny's hanky drawer, and among my all-time favourite beauty smells.

The Little Round Pot franchise has been expanded over the years to include creme blushers that are among the very best at any price, and the packaging updated from rococo cherub design cardboard to chintzy floral tin, to gold-stamped coloured Bakelite (the packaging I grew up with), and the more convenient mirrored snap-compact we see today. But what has remained throughout is the chubby, tactile shape and moreish shade line-up that make Bourjois Little Round Pots the kind of rainy lunchtime purchase that can keep a girl going until clock-out.

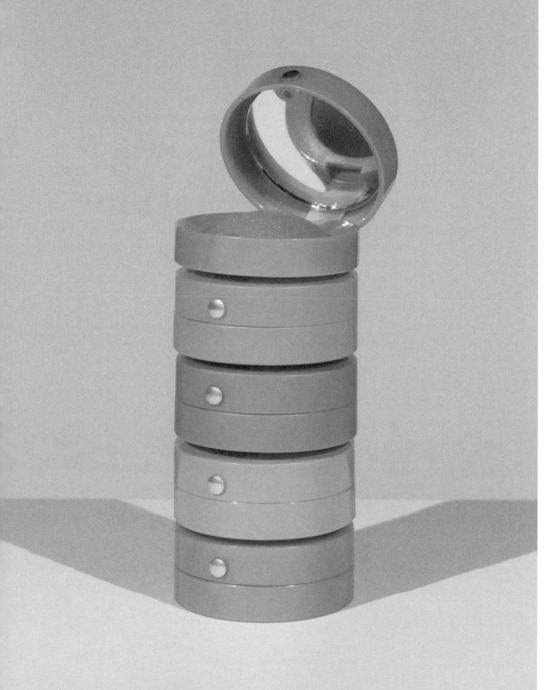

I must give props to Evian for somehow making a beauty icon of an almost laughably unnecessary product, but then the entire bottled water industry is based on turning a relatively free resource into a marketable commodity, so I guess popping water into an aerosol in the name of beauty was a fairly short leap for them to make. Yes, I am deeply cynical but yes, I am also no more immune to the hype than the next person. There was a time in my life when an Evian Brumisateur was all my heart desired. Magazines of the 1980s were always singing its praises, and if you were the kind of person who hoovered up every interview with make-up artists and beauty editors, you soon realised that this large can of water was in every industry kitbag.

Why? It's a good question. The assertion by beauty professionals was that it 'set' make-up in place, though I've never personally found any evidence that this could be true, even over old-fashioned make-up formulas. It was also used to 'freshen' skin at the start of photo shoots, which is valid, if one has no access to a tap and an empty spray bottle, which admittedly were not as commonly available, and much less fine in the eighties (gardening sprays were more of a shower than a spritz). Where I can see the use for a Brumisateur is if you are working in some remote location, where cold water is scarce (the tin can tends to keep the water cooler), or if you are easily overheated – like in menopause – and you want something cooling and chemical-free in your handbag that won't potentially cause any irritation.

In any case, Evian Brumisateur was successful in making itself a hugely desirable product, and in securing its place in every beauty junkie's arsenal. I associate its packaging with the cluttered make-up table on countless photo shoots and filming sets and absolutely will concede that it launched an entire beauty category of facial spritzers, now a feature in most skincare brands with the addition of plant extracts, hyaluronic acid, glycerin and so on. I've also no doubt the dubious myth that a final spray of water locks make-up in place went on to inspire the development of true make-up fixing sprays like those by Urban Decay, MAC, NYX, Clarins and many others. But mostly I still see Evian's original as little more than a status symbol born in an era obsessed with acquiring them. As with our obsession with buying wasteful plastic bottles of water in safe and plentiful supply from our own kitchen taps, I often think that future generations will look at Evian Brumisateur and wonder if ours had temporarily taken leave of its senses.

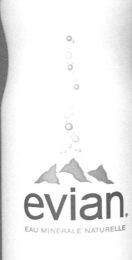

Much like prawns, gin and bracelets, Benefit Benetint is something that looks so completely up my street, and yet, however persistently I try, I just can't get onboard. My skin is too dry and too thirsty for this liquid rose-petal lip and cheek stain and so it sinks in well before I can blend it, and there it remains, like a clumsy Malbec spill on a white shag pile. On normals and oilies, Benetint is beautiful – but this isn't the only reason I'm able to love it. Sometimes one quirky, interesting product can create enough mystique and ecstatic word of mouth, that it alone has the power to launch an empire – and never has that been more pleasingly demonstrated than here.

In 1977 an exotic dancer entered the tiny San Francisco beauty boutique of twins Jean and Jane Ford, and asked for something to stain her nipples (I do so enjoy hearing of a beauty gripe even I'd never considered), making them bright, perky and noticeable throughout a long show on a dark stage. The sisters took up the gauntlet and began experimenting in their kitchen, steaming real rose petals to create a deep, vivid red liquor to stain the skin. The liquid was poured in a tiny cork-stoppered glass bottle, hand-labelled with a naive line drawing of a single bloom, named 'Rose Tint' and delivered to the dancer. Needless to say, it was enthusiastically received, applied more widely than on the nips, and soon dozens of San Franciscan women wanted in.

Gradually, Benefit took off, arriving in the UK in the late nineties, where just a tiny handful of products were sold at Harrods. The press were captivated, the buzz about the by then repackaged and renamed Benetint in particular was huge. Now, Benefit is one of Britain's top five bestselling colour brands. Some of their products are superb: they are particularly good at brows, bronzers and highlighters, but that original nipple tint remains its hero. When brushed onto the right skin and rubbed in with fingertips, it adds a pretty, effortless rose flush straight out of a Pre-Raphaelite watercolour that, sadly, I can only admire second-hand.

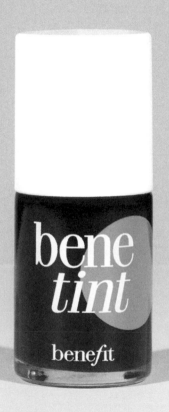

I don't know if you've ever sat in a hairdresser's salon and witnessed your stylist find themselves temporarily unable to locate his or her Mason Pearson hairbrush, but I have on several occasions and can assure you it's not pretty. Woe betide any chancer who attempted to make off with it. This is because a Mason Pearson rubber cushion brush remains, over 200 years after its original invention, the gold standard throughout the hairdressing world, with each owner feeling as attached to theirs as a chef to her favourite paring knife. I feel similarly about my own cherished brushes.

I encountered my first Mason Pearson at around six years old, when my aunt came to stay from London with a girlfriend who unpacked a large Mason Pearson and placed it ceremoniously on my tiny dressing table next to her Z-bed. Before then, I'd thought that hairbrushes were two quid jobs from the corner shop or chemist and associated them with tortuous and tear-filled detangling sessions in front of the fire – so fraught that my father once felt a yellow plastic handle, defeated by a knot as unyielding as a boulder, snap clean in half in my hair and sort of dangle, like Fay Wray in King Kong's clutches. The Mason Pearson was different. Like the Mary Poppins of hairbrushes, it was firm, sturdy and no-nonsense but kind, modest and uncommonly elegant. Sadly, there was no way a family like ours could ever spend a week's grocery money on a hairbrush, and so I had to wait until adulthood, when I was earning my own money and found myself in a traditional chemist in Mayfair ostensibly looking for Nurofen. That same 19-year-old 'Handy' sized Mason Pearson is still on my dressing table today, nobly doing its job, while an 8-year-old 'Pocket' size lives permanently in my handbag.

It's endlessly satisfying to me that in an age of ceramic-barrelled, laser-cut, heated and rotating contraptions, this high-quality British-made icon prevails. Anyone who's ever owned a Mason Pearson will know why. The weighty plastic handle (or a wooden one if you're a purist – they're still available on some models) feels smooth and solid in the hand, the bristles (natural bristle for fine hair, a bristle and nylon mix for normal hair, nylon bristles for thick and curly hair) glide through locks like a spoon through cream, gently massaging the scalp to dislodge dirt and distribute natural oils down the shaft, thus eliminating frizz. It backcombs brilliantly, neither scratches nor pulls, tames hair without causing static, and dries fringes or bangs better than anything (just pull the brush back and forth across your forehead while the dryer nozzle points downward). The Mason Pearson can also be used on children's hair (I invariably buy the child's size as christening gifts) without them wailing from bath to bedtime. The brush itself is extremely easy – and satisfying – to clean with a sturdy wide-toothed comb.

Of course, any Mason Pearson owner would be lying if they claimed not to have been drawn, at least in part, to its heirloom-worthy looks. The signature gold-blocked 'Dark Ruby' (black on first glance, a gemstone red when held up to the light) handle and orange rubber cushion make it utilitarian but elegant, and recognisable the world over. And despite the incomparability of the Mason Pearson, so many are still trying to copy it, even marking up the already painful price point. It's wholly unseemly and I reject them utterly.

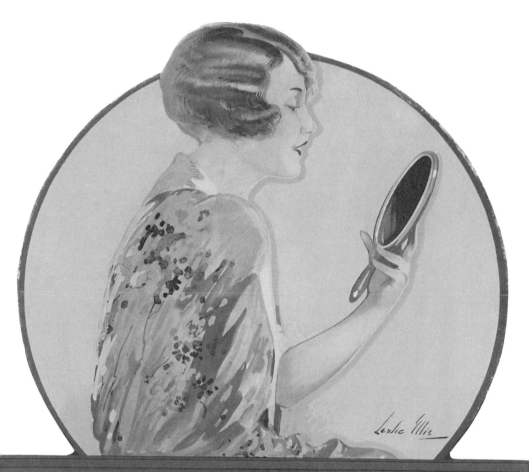

Well Brushed Hair is Beautiful Hair

MASON PEARSON
HAIR BRUSH

Let's be perfectly honest, there's nothing exceptional or special about Herbal Essences shampoo and conditioner. They smell rather lovely, they do the job perfectly well, they come at a great price point, can be bought anywhere and their name sounds pleasingly like a reggae compilation album circa 1973. What makes them iconic is a single marketing campaign, conceived as a do-or-die last-chance saloon for a tired-looking haircare franchise at Clairol, at a time when Herbal Essences was a generic family haircare brand with no USP to speak of. By the late 1990s, beauty brands using natural plant extracts were a dime to a dozen, many of them doing it more thoroughly and more authentically. Herbal Essences had always been marketed at everyone, and thereby appealed to no one.

Ad execs decided to give the brand a boot up the backside with a campaign zoning in on women rather than the entire family. Borrowing heavily from Nora Ephron's *When Harry Met Sally,* the groundbreaking new campaign featured women, standing alone in the shower, loudly climaxing as they lathered up with Herbal Essences shampoo, suggesting that this run-of-the-mill brand was far from an unremarkable, stuffy seventies relic, but a 'totally orgasmic' experience. The ads were pretty tame – cheeky rather than softly pornographic – but for a generation of women who'd grown up in token sex education classes without ever hearing mention of the female orgasm, they represented a sea-change in middle-of-the-road beauty advertising and marketing. Herbal Essences was no longer about the dutiful housewife leaning over the bath to wash her children's hair while a chicken roasted in the oven, it was a brand for women and recognised their need for 'me time' (I promise I will never use this mortifying expression again). Of course, the campaign rather overstated the product's effects – unless a woman was to be more imaginative with the water hose, a shower with Herbal Essences was unlikely to yield greater results than cleaner hair. And it's true that after we became inured to the original gimmick, and other brands pushed the envelope further, Clairol was back to square one. We now lived in a world where reality TV stars had sex on telly and defecated in front of six hidden cameras.

In the mid-noughties, P&G, having acquired Clairol, redesigned and relaunched Herbal Essences, scrapping the pastel bottles and Totally Orgasmic Experience in favour of lurid brights and a red carpet-wannabe message. These effects were also short-lived. A few years later, P&G rightly went back to the old, by now iconic bottles and smells. Where that leaves Herbal Essences is anyone's guess. Where it perhaps leaves women is with little more than sexual frustration and a pleasant, vaguely chemical herbal scent.

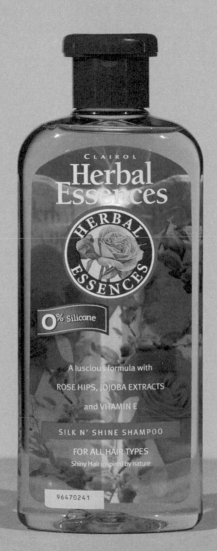

Old Spice Original, launched in 1938, is the smell from the backseat of my grandad's brown Austin Allegro as he drove me to Little Chef for the giddy treat of jumbo cod, chips, banana split and a free lollipop for clearing my plate. Its warm, not-too-strong but lasting spiciness is the smell of day trips to Tenby, of candy-stripe brushed flannel sheets from the market, of a tiny metalwork room made from a cubby-hole under the stairs. It's the smell of the armchair where we took Sunday naps during the rugby, had cuddles and belly laughs in front of Victoria Wood's *As Seen On TV*, where my grandad sat patiently as I stood on a stool behind him, tying bows, plaits, jewels and fancy clips in his white hair, not giving a damn if he had to answer the door for the postman.

Old Spice is the scent of him trying to teach me long division when everyone else had long ago lost patience, of very gentle flirting with the checkout ladies at Kwiksave, of seemingly endless chats with every Indian and Pakistani immigrant in Blackwood to practise his beloved Urdu and Burmese learned during the Second World War in Burma. It's the smell that filled a silent room whenever I asked what had happened to his friends there. Old Spice is the smell of his old shirt worn over my ra-ra dress to wash the car, of well-thumbed Robert Ludlum novels, of huge cotton handkerchiefs, of an often empty wallet, of the green zip-up anorak bought via twenty weekly payments from the Peter Craig catalogue. Old Spice was there when J.R. Ewing was shot, when I first saw Madonna on *Top of the Pops*, when the miners went back to work and when we sat under blankets at military tattoos, both of us weeping like newborns. Its absence was felt acutely when I last saw his face, eyes closed in the room of a hospice; when I got married and when my babies were born.

Clearly, I'm too sentimental about Old Spice for my opinion to be truly objective, but unlike so many other scents of my youth, I believe Old Spice Original (not its newer, nastier incarnations) is still a gorgeous fragrance in its own right. It's neither ironic nor retro, just a wholly pleasant blend of nutmeg, cinnamon, clove, star anise, exotic jasmine, warm vanilla and sweet geranium, packaged in one of the most beautiful perfume bottles of all time. For the world's bestselling mass-market fragrance, and an indisputable beauty and grooming icon, Old Spice Original still feels like a very unique and personal affair. I revere it for many reasons, but not least because, as its early ad campaign asserted, 'You probably wouldn't be here if your grandfather hadn't worn Old Spice'.

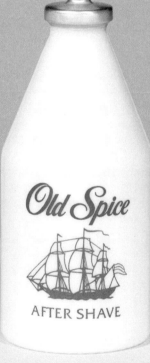

I give huge credit to OPI for creating a polish that in many ways has become as standard a red as that of London buses, award season carpets, Welsh Guards, the stripes on American flags and the coats on Chelsea Pensioners. It is consistently at number one across OPI's shades and, cumulatively, is officially the brand's bestselling lacquer of all time. For a polish launched as late as 1999, I'm Not Really a Waitress has certainly got around. Apart from being the go-to red for TV and film make-up artists who love its dense, multi-dimensional finish (it shows up really well on camera without stealing the scene), I'm Not Really a Waitress has featured as the $16,000 question on the US version of *Who Wants to Be a Millionaire*, been used as the colour reference point for a red Dell laptop and has won the Reader's Choice Favourite Nail Colour Award in *Allure* magazine a staggering nine years on the skip. The seal on its iconic status: the *Urban Dictionary* even recognises I'm Not Really a Waitress as 'The specific color of red nail polish that is used in countless movies and commercials for its sheer mass appeal'.

I agree that the key to its success is that I'm Not Really a Waitress truly looks good on everyone, and with everything. It's a ruby slippers red that flatters black, brown, yellow, pink and white skins equally, and layers very well for greater depth. It looks expensive and neat, leaving nails like the bonnet of a metallic red Porsche. The sparkling – but not glittery – finish makes it glamorous enough for parties (it's my default Christmas polish – so festive and jolly) but restrained enough for work meetings. The unforgettable if slightly annoying name also helps. Launched originally for OPI's Hollywood Collection, the name – typical of the brand's quirky wordplay – is a homage to wannabe movie stars making rent by waiting tables while they wait for their big break. And so it's fitting, really, that I'm Not Really a Waitress has ended up making so many uncredited appearances in big Hollywood blockbusters.

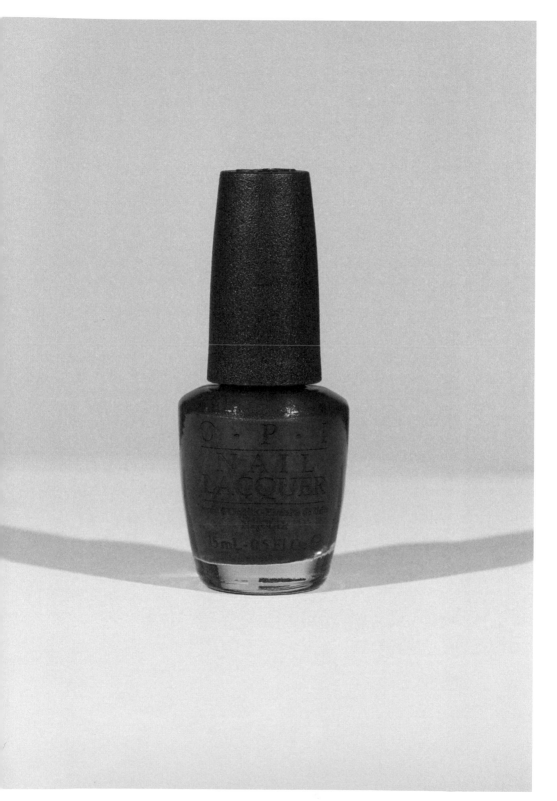

I'm sent every conceivable hair product, including luxury shampoos costing upwards of £30, but there are times when nothing hits the spot like a two quid bottle of Pantene. There's something about its mass-market chemical fragrance that has been weirdly sexy to me from the first time I encountered it in the 1980s, then allowing me to overlook its pretty revolting, albeit hugely successful, advertising slogan of 'Don't hate me because I'm beautiful'. Everyone used Pantene in those days (I once found myself in a famous supermodel's bathroom and, not entirely without effort, discovered several Pantene bottles on the go). Personally, it was never my favourite shampoo and isn't now. But it's certainly more than serviceable, especially over periods of four to five weeks' use (after that, it can be prone to causing build-up and lankness and will need to be swapped for a bit – unless you're using the new-ish silicone-free version, where the problem is largely eradicated).

There's more to Pantene than shampoo and conditioner, though, of course. The entire brand is based on the discovery in the 1940s by scientists at Swiss drug company Hoffmann-La Roche, that panthenol, a pro-vitamin of B5, had 'healing effects' on damaged hair. The Pantene brand – much posher in those days – was born and today (under the different ownership of P&G) there are dozens of hair conditioning products under its umbrella: decent masks, hairsprays and mousses for every hair type, and the world's first 2-in-1 shampoo and conditioner (it was not, contrary to assumptions, Vidal Sassoon's Wash & Go), all of them built around the same key ingredient of panthenol. Perhaps more relevant to my interests is the continuity throughout the line of that same unmistakable fragrance. It has the sweet, addictive, unisex scent I now think of as the generic smell of 'clean hair'. I can't imagine there'll ever be a time I no longer crave it.

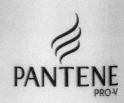

When the SK-II brand arrived in Britain in the late 1990s, packaged in minimalist glass bottles and tubes, with little to no enclosed information, at an almost unprecedented price point, I'm afraid I largely ignored it on the basis that it seemed impenetrable and to fancy itself a bit too much. A few years later, make-up legend Mary Greenwell told me that her regular client Cate Blanchett absolutely swore by it and so, given that Blanchett has skin like vellum, it seemed mad not to at least give it a whirl. Despite my former misgivings, I loved it and was newly intrigued by its philosophy. I won't tell it as wistfully nor as reverently as intended, but here goes: a little over thirty years ago, scientists observed that elderly workers in Japanese sake breweries had wrinkled faces but astonishingly soft, youthful, line-free hands. They analysed the fermentation liquid with which the workers were in constant physical contact, and after countless tests, they found the answer in a unique yeast strain they named Pitera. The ingredient, rich in over fifty minerals, organic acids, vitamins and amino acids, would form the basis of every product in SK-II, a new luxury anti-ageing skincare brand.

But in hindsight, the even bigger story was in the Japanese skincare rituals SK-II demanded. This was not your traditional Western cleanse, tone, moisturise-type deal. The two-step SK-II cleansing ritual alone took longer. What followed it was the cornerstone of the entire SK-II philosophy: Facial Treatment Essence. This is a treatment liquid (not a toner) containing over 90 per cent pure Pitera, applied directly to clean skin with either fingertips or a cotton disc. It was the first of its kind, and undoubtedly inspired the huge number of Japanese-style treatment essences we see in the West today. The act of double cleansing (not that I think it particularly necessary myself) is now the gold standard for many skincare fans, and the multi-step morning and night ritual is regarded by many as a perfectly normal and pleasurable way to spend the best part of an hour. For better or worse, SK-II certainly helped nudge us eastwards.

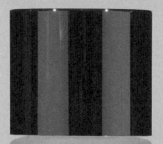

It's a bit odd, when you think about it, for a company's two best known products to be a razor – and a pen. But such unlikely portfolio-mates make a lot more sense when you consider their common defining feature: cheap chuckability. Bic's pens arrived first – a fabulous moment in company history coming after the war when Mr Bic (actually Marcel Bich) pleasingly bought the patent for the ballpoint pen from Mr Biro. Bich improved the design of the pen while dramatically lowering the price through mass production, and Bic's brand value was born.

So when the company launched the iconic white and orange plastic disposable razor in 1975, it wasn't the continuation of a heritage brand, the product of time-served artisans who'd been hand-crafting steel blades since the court of Louis XIV. It was a shrewd move by a company who knew how to make cheap stuff out of plastic and had spotted a way to make shaving one step less fiddly. Up to that point, cartridges had evolved to become both safer and more easily exchanged, but Bic's disposable razor was the first that invited the user to bin the entire device. A minimalist design classic, the featureless T of the Bic razor offers no comfortable grip, no reassuring weight, no decoration.

But long superseded as it may be by multiple blades, multi-directional tilting heads and gel strips (and my legs certainly prefer them to a common Bic), there's still an undoubted appeal to a razor you can buy in big bags like potatoes, grab one as needed, use once and throw away with minimal guilt. The more expensive and many-featured the modern blade, the greater the obligation to rinse and reuse, to tease out stubborn shavings from between the blades, to ignore the faded aloe strip and convince yourself there're still two good shaves in it. Bic's one-shave stand was revolutionary, its convenience for sleepovers, holidays and pre-payday frugality, deathless. The disposable razor is rightly considered not only a beauty icon, but one of the greatest single inventions of all time.

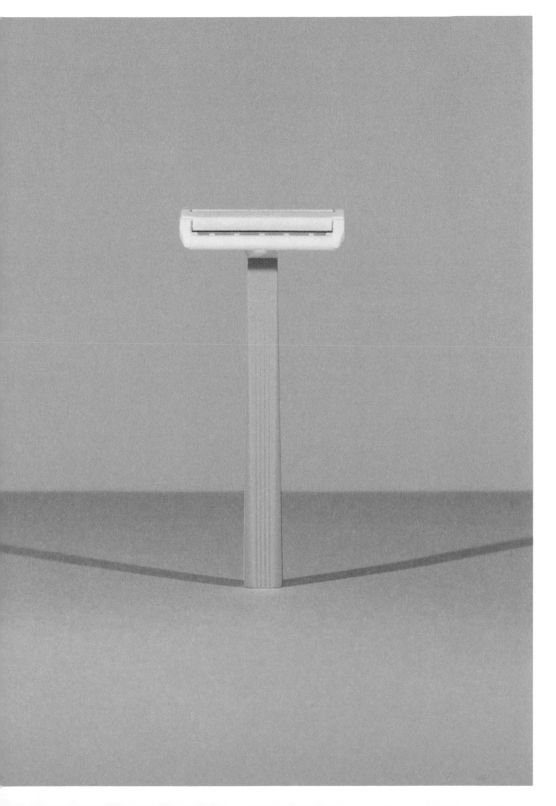

It seems that the more expensive and luxurious the skincare product I recommend (and I do so sparingly and with a sense of responsibility) in my journalism, the more likely it is for some wearyingly furious person to crash into my Twitter feed and tell me that her granny died at 109, with not a single wrinkle on her face, all thanks to carbolic soap and a daily spread of good old-fashioned Nivea Creme. This pure white multi-purpose moisturiser (named Nivea after the Latin word for snow), essentially unchanged for over a hundred years, has become the sort of figurehead for unfussy, no-nonsense beauty, devoid of vanity or frippery, the kind of unpretentious preparation that makes fools of the competition and its users. This, as well as being absurd – there's nothing wrong with spending your own money on whatever you like – also rather sells Nivea short, because it was quite the cutting-edge skincare in its day and as a brand has continued to innovate ever since.

Nivea (part of the Beiersdorf company from day one) was the first mass-produced stable oil- and-water-based cream and remained the company's sole product for many years, but from the Second World War onwards the brand rolled out many great products like body lotion, shaving cream, oil, shampoo and, later, the excellent male grooming, anti-ageing and suncare ranges we see today (I go nowhere in summer without Nivea's ingenious handbag-sized tube of SPF30). But far from feeling irked by the anti-beauty brigade's weapon of choice, I am cheered by the original Nivea Creme's continued existence. It's a lovely, sturdy little product for ungreasily moisturising and softening dry hands, arms, legs and feet. If you suffer no adverse effects from paraffin derivatives, there's nothing to stop you wearing it on your face (the velvety finish makes for a surprisingly decent make-up base, as it happens). And despite Nivea Creme's reputation for simplicity, it has perhaps the most beautiful fragrance on all the high street. It smells clean, slightly beeswaxy and super feminine – very similar, in fact, to Nina Ricci's L'Air du Temps, only for less than the price of a Sunday newspaper.

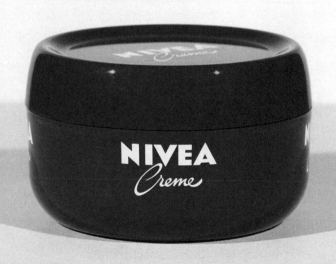

My love of this product is merely notional, since I don't recall ever having it in the house as a child, despite two babies arriving after me. Johnson's baby shampoo – the first shampoo to utilise amphoretic cleansing agents, so gentle that they lightly cleaned without stinging the eyes – seemed like something owned by the kind of family who probably had a purpose-decorated nursery, a wallpaper border to match the Moses basket, a savings account opened and a school place lined up for a newborn. It wasn't for big chaotic families like ours, prone to bathing babies in the kitchen sink, complete with Fairy Liquid bubble beard and reachable access to the bread knife.

It was decades later that I finally used No More Tears to wash my make-up brushes, the popular opinion being that it didn't strip and dry out the bristles. I'm no longer convinced that it's the best substance for such a job (I use any non-moisturising shampoo that happens to be in the shower), since No More Tears' very mild cleansing action is aimed at babies who are barely dirty to begin with, never mind caked in old foundation and powder, but it's true that if your brushes are used rarely or lightly, or your hair is pretty clean, then No More Tears will spruce up hairs nicely. The bright yellow formula, as you might expect, rinses quickly and smells deliciously of babies – sweet, comforting and cosy – and the pebble-shaped bottle is pleasingly unmodernised.

I bought some in readiness for my first baby, when just owning the right supplies made me feel in control, and whenever I used it I momentarily felt like a proper mum despite the fact that I was entirely at sea. And maybe that is exactly why Johnson's No More Tears baby shampoo has been an unwavering, deeply loved icon since 1936. When the disorientating, confusing, guilt-ridden and anxious, albeit ultimately wonderful, experience of motherhood strikes, it stands nobly by the side of the bath, as reassuringly experienced as a nanny, making one feel as though everything will be okay.

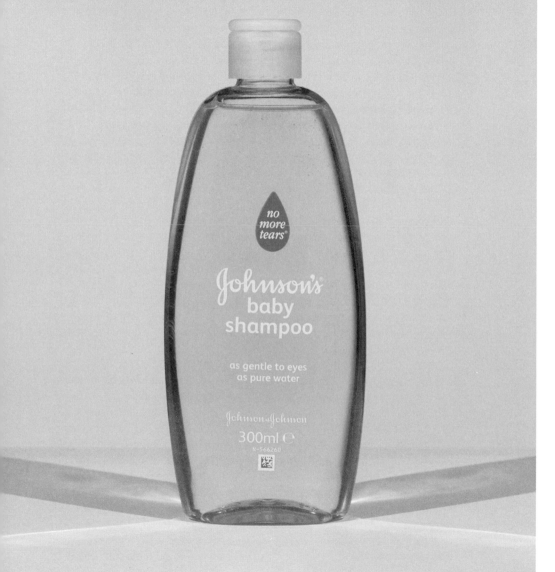

If I had a penny for every time someone sidled up to me at a function, found out what I do, and asked me, 'Is Crème de la Mer really worth all that money?', then I'd have enough cash to swim in the stuff. The expectation is that I'll say either that this super-expensive moisturiser is miraculous and life-changing, or that it's rubbish and dishonest (and you'll find plenty of reviews online of people taking one of these two extreme positions). The reality, for me at least, is a tad more nuanced. Crème de la Mer was invented over fifty years ago by aerospace physicist Dr Max Huber, after he'd suffered burns in a laboratory accident and wanted to improve his scarred, damaged skin. He became obsessed with the way natural sea kelp retained moisture and regenerated itself and hand-harvested and fermented supplies for his experiments. He turned the fermented kelp into what he nicknamed 'Miracle Broth', combined it with simple skincare ingredients for minimal irritation, and Crème de la Mer was born. It's a romantic story, but in beauty those are ten a penny.

What people really want to know is if it works. For me, I have to say in all honesty that it broadly does. My super-dry skin looks better when I use it. People invariably tell me I look well by the time I'm a third of the way into a jar. On the rare occasions I've experienced an allergic reaction to something else I've been testing, an instant switchover to Crème de la Mer (with Clarins SOS serum underneath) has metaphorically put out the fire in days. Friends who've undergone chemo tell me with utter conviction that it's all their skin could tolerate at the height of related dryness and sensitivity (though I am certain some people would react to the inclusion of eucalyptus oil). I'm sure many would argue convincingly that this is psychosomatic, but I personally don't think that matters in the least (if, God forbid, I'm ever seriously ill, I'll want things that make me feel nice as much as I'll want things that make me feel better, and woe betide anyone who preachily shoves Vaseline under my nose and tells me to use that instead).

Personally, I use this simple, uncomplicated, pleasurable cream as a skin saver when things go pear-shaped, not as a daily moisturiser, and certainly not as an anti-ageing cream. I suggest people should manage their expectations on that score – this is not a wrinkle cream, or an exfoliant, or an antioxidant of any remarkable merit. It's a softening, soothing, rich, buttery moisturiser that looks and feels luxurious. You can certainly do as well for much less money and those with oily or combination skin are unlikely to find the original Crème suits them (bafflingly, it contains mineral oil. Some of the other products in the range, like the oil, do not). But nonetheless Crème de la Mer is an icon. Its launch, cachet and subsequent success absolutely marked a sea change in skincare – perhaps an unwelcome one, since in terms of exclusivity and high price point, it's now far from unique – and, I think, helped spark an increased public interest in skincare. 'It-creams' (a term invented by the media for Crème de la Mer, but applied at one time to any cream over £50 – oh, but were that still exceptional) now exist in the portfolio of almost every luxury brand, and yet truly there is still no product more coveted, more intriguing to the average consumer after all these years, than Crème. So there is my answer. Imagine how many polite party-goers wish they'd never asked.

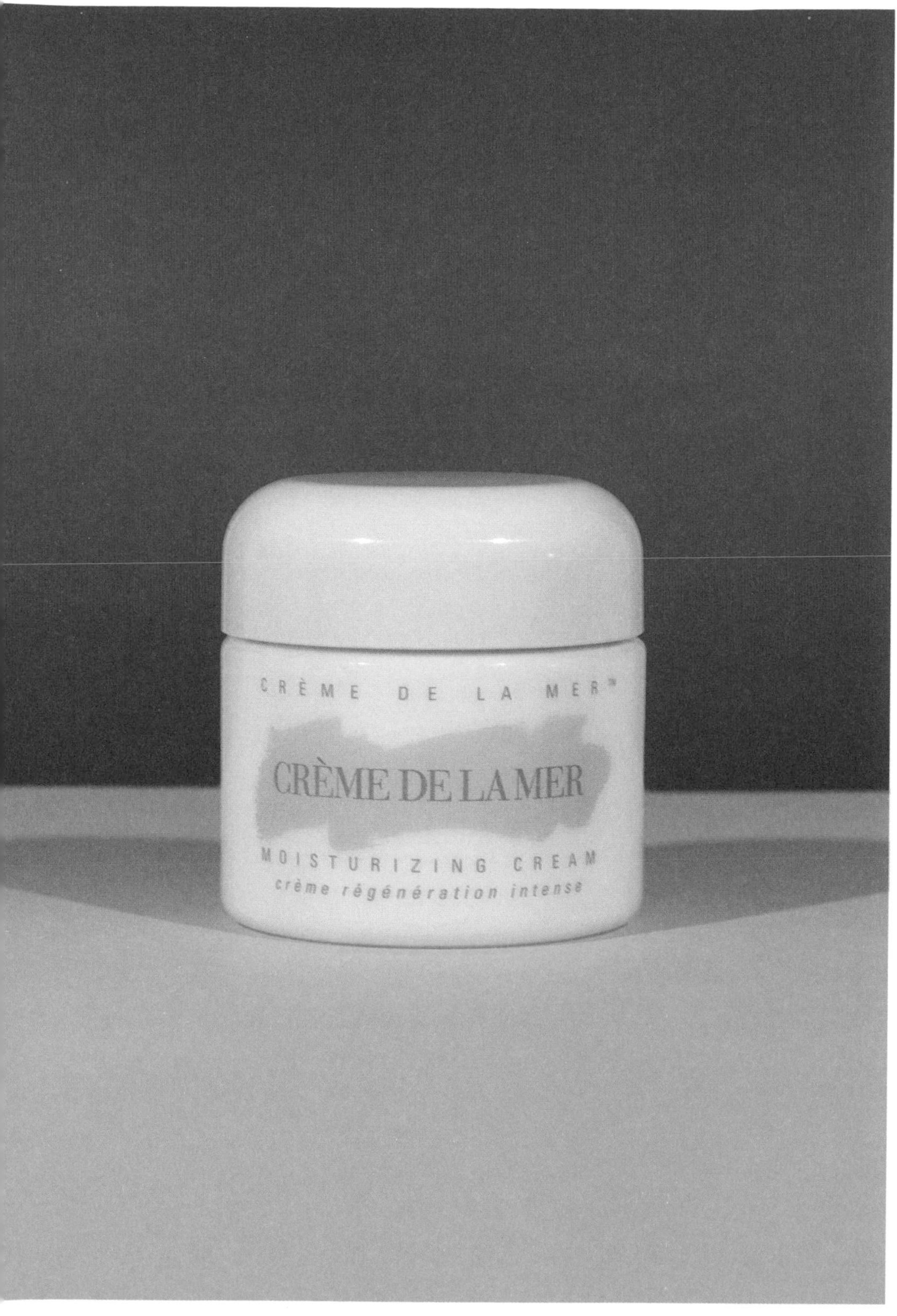

I knew about Head & Shoulders before I even knew what dandruff was. The weird vase-shaped bottle lived around our bath and on TV commercials featuring brooding male models slowly raking their side partings to reveal for the camera an infestation of props department snow. They'd then lather one side of their scalp with Head & Shoulders, the other with a generic shampoo, the miraculous results shown on split-screen TV. It wasn't until secondary school, and I discovered the pitfalls of wearing the regulation black cardigan, that I realised why – a few Timotei fanciers aside – seemingly everyone used Head & Shoulders. And it's a credit to P&G's clever marketing that a potentially embarrassing problem like dandruff became so normalised that the shampoo was such an accepted mainstream beauty staple. Celebrities such as Jeff Daniels, Ulrika Jonsson, Sofia Vergara, Jenson Button and now premiership goalkeeper Joe Hart have all cheerfully cashed a cheque regardless of the inherent implication they have scalp fungus. And why not?

Head & Shoulders is still the world's bestselling shampoo, still has a strong, slightly chalky whiff of big box washing powder, and to give credit where it's most due, it still works – with a couple of caveats. Head & Shoulders uses zinc pyrithione to control the levels of micro-organisms on the scalp (the most common form of dandruff comes from yeast growing in skin sebum) and so can only do its job for as long as you're using it. If you stop, or dramatically cut down, your dandruff will return. And back to my school cardigan: I soon found that Head & Shoulders had little or no effect on me, because I didn't have traditional dandruff from oiliness and sebum. I just had a dry scalp. If you're the same, seek out a shampoo – preferably sulphate-free – for this specific problem and treat your scalp to the odd olive oil massage the night before shampooing. You'll see much lighter snowfall.

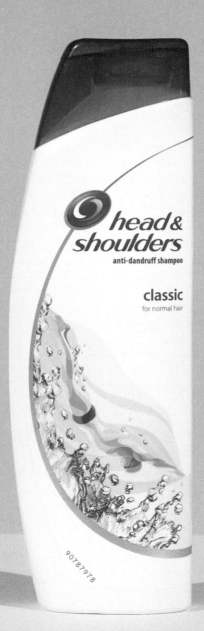

I'm sure I've mentioned it previously, but I hate most mascaras. Which is an inconvenience if you'd sooner saw off your big toe than never wear it again. My issue with it is that it's not good enough. I so often despair of how little progress the industry has made over the years in developing just one mascara that does everything I want: separate, curl, define, darken, thicken, lengthen, lift, stay, remove. On shoots, make-up artists will invariably use several different mascaras on just one model. Maybe a Maybelline to build up, a little Tom Ford to kick out at the sides, some MAC Gigablack to really blacken, some Kevyn Aucoin tubing to lock the whole thing down ... Now brands are pushing this whole (potentially very lucrative) mascara portfolio nonsense, but really, who on earth has the time? I'm lucky to get two coats on between Brighton and Hayward's Heath, never mind rustle around for different wands for different jobs.

But what I've found, time and time again, when looking into the make-up bags of industry figures as pushed for time and space as the rest of us, is this. When it comes to mascara, most experts will agree that Lancôme is a safe pair of hands. They know their mascara better than almost anyone and for a number of years were head and shoulders above the competition. They make no attempt at subtlety (natural-looking mascaras are the chocolate teapot of beauty), but go all out for the kind of fluttery, separated and thickened lashes most of us desire. The formula of Hypnôse is neither wet and messy, nor dry and spiky. It stays fresh for longer, the expertly designed brush coats each and every lash perfectly. The black is real black, not some insipid shade the colour of a faded sock. It is probably the best we have.

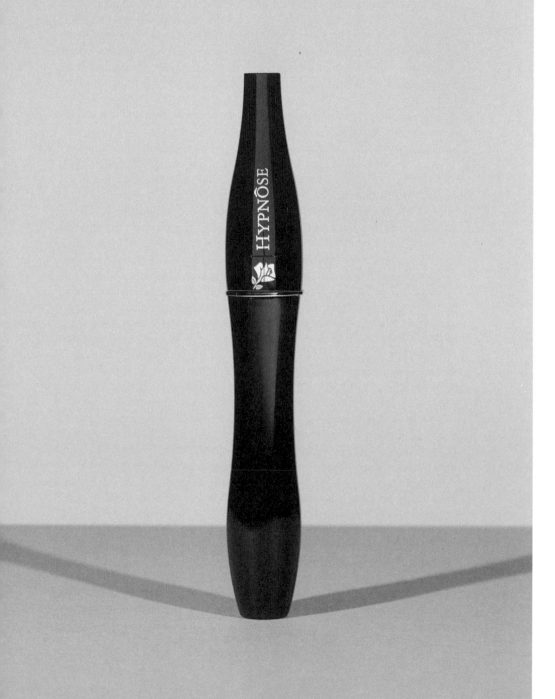

In terms of iconography, Vaseline is the Campbell's soup tin, Coke can or Brillo pad box of beauty. Practically everyone owns it, and those who don't could readily identify its blue-capped jar – and probably list at least five uses for its contents, some of them downright filthy. Robert Augustus Chesebrough, a 22-year-old British chemist, could not have conceived of such success when he invented Vaseline by chance in 1859. He was visiting a Pennsylvania town where petroleum had recently been discovered. He became intrigued by the by-product of the oil-drilling process and observed the oil workers rubbing drill residue into their cuts and burns to heal them. Inspired, he triple-distilled it, cleaning out impurities (Vaseline is still the only petroleum jelly that goes through this process), perfecting the formula over ten years. He then opened a factory in New York and got on his horse and cart to sell his 'Wonder Jelly' to the public (mainly by burning himself with acid before an audience, then smearing the wound with it, like some sort of lunatic).

It was a massive success. He renamed it, expanded his distribution, and soon found himself at the helm of a large beauty brand, growing by the month. His petroleum jelly was taken by explorers on the first successful expedition to the North Pole (on account of it not freezing), was made standard issue for US soldiers in the trenches of the First World War, coated special healing gauze for use on the front line during the Second World War, and was stocked in both hospitals and home first-aid kits. A tub of Vaseline is sold every thirty-nine seconds somewhere in the world, and is utilised in a vast petroleum-based product range. Poured into a tin it becomes Vaseline Lip Therapy, the world's biggest lip brand. Whipped with glycerin into lotion, it becomes Vaseline Intensive Care Lotion, the first port of call for many dry skin sufferers. In beauty alone, it has endless applications. It slicks down unruly brows, adds sheen to cheekbones, mixes with any powder to become coloured gloss, adds shine to legs, removes old glue from false lashes, blends with sugar to act as a lip scrub, diverts self-tan headed for dry spots, and lines cuticles to prevent nail polish migration. It is never missing from photo shoots, where in the past it even greased up camera lenses to give film stars a misty, otherworldly glow.

I myself am not the biggest fan of paraffins and mineral oil in expensive products (although my skin doesn't particularly object to them). I believe that brands expecting you to spend big bucks on skincare should first dig deep into their own pockets and use much nicer plant oils that won't cause breakouts. But in products as cheap as Vaseline, I'm more charitable, if not a particularly committed user myself. There's an honesty here. What you see is what you get – a cheap, greasy petroleum jelly that fulfils its promise to temporarily moisturise, lubricate and seal. It is deeply unpretentious, egalitarian, often appropriate and much loved by millions. In my view, there are now far better products for each one of its uses. But none that do all of them at once, and certainly none as truly iconic.

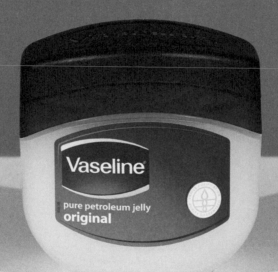

In the early 1900s T.L. Williams made, from dyes and Vaseline, a mascara for his little sister Maybel, and called it Lash-Brow-Ine. The solid, cake formula was to name and launch the Maybelline brand, but its enduring status as the high street/drugstore mascara specialist came via Great Lash in 1971. If I was asked to close my eyes and think of a mascara, I'd see the gaudy hot pink and lurid green of Great Lash. Its iconic status is in part down to this packaging (virtually unchanged since launch), so far along the trashy and kitsch continuum that it emerges completely fabulous at the other end. But there's more about Great Lash than an instantly recognisable tube. It is the one mascara one unfailingly sees on photo shoots, television make-up room tables or film sets.

There are several reasons for this: it's proper, opaque, dark soot-black, not that semi-transparent dirty puddle shade so woefully common in cheaper mascaras. Also, the brush (any good mascara is a 50/50 combination of formula and brush shape) can be manoeuvred into the deepest set eyes, along even the puniest lashes to give excellent definition. Its finish is slightly wet-looking, its formula is thin enough to be layered ad infinitum like mattresses atop the princess's pea, until lashes are thick and spiky, like sixties Twiggy's. It doesn't go crunchy, dry or flake onto cheeks.

It isn't the mascara I unfailingly turn to by any means (it doesn't quickly give the dramatic, kittenish lashes so many of us crave, and it smudges on me – but then so do 95 per cent of all mascaras), but undeniably it represents a starting point for most of what came after. The original cake may be long gone, but Great Lash, along with Full 'n' Soft (a more natural-looking mascara, woefully unavailable in the UK – do try it if ever Stateside), remain, as do various Great Lash spin-offs, including a waterproof formula. I'm glad original Great Lash remains relatively untouched, as it should.

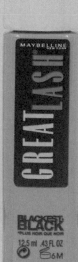

I could have chosen any one of a handful of iconic products from cool New York apothecary brand Kiehl's. Creme With Silk Groom, the hairstyling cream so loved by session hairdressers to give sleek, ungreasy definition to shorter styles and crazy curls, perhaps (not that I have ever in my life got to grips with it). Or Blue Astringent Herbal Lotion, a potent toner that makes you momentarily brace. Certainly Kiehl's lip balm qualifies easily, since so many beauty fans, myself included, made pilgrimages to London's Liberty or Harvey Nichols to pick up a tube before Kiehl's was on every high street. But from all of Kiehl's products, I've concluded that the true icon is Creme de Corps, the celebrated cocoa butter and sesame oil body cream, loved for its richness and superior moisturising on very dry skin.

This thick, custardy cream, smelling weirdly, but pleasingly, like the paint in a primary school craft lesson, was among the first products developed by Irving Morse, the Russian-Jewish immigrant who bought the original East Village Kiehl's apothecary-style store in 1921. It has remained a Kiehl's bestseller ever since. It's a fairly uncompromising product that relies on word of mouth among dry and sensitive skin sufferers. Even on the thirstiest skins, rubbing it in can be like kneading dough, and if you're sitting on a nice white towel at the time, you can expect it to be stained temporarily with crème brûlée smears and blotches (it's only the beta carotene and nothing more sinister). But the results are fabulous: skin is sort of cocooned in rich moisture, not greasy and grubby-feeling. It's very good at giving shins an even, very slightly shiny finish, and at improving the look of blotchy upper arms. It's great for post-tattoo healing and on babies and children with eczema and other dry skin conditions (oh, that I'd had Creme de Corps as a kid). It's the loveliest product to slather thickly on post-bath skin, then get into clean pyjamas and a freshly made bed, phone on divert, massive mug of tea and a remote control at one's side.

There's a whipped version in a tub, though I've had much less success with it. It has a more matte finish but starts to bobble and peel away if you massage too hard. There's a lighter version too, though I feel it rather misses the point of Creme de Corps, which is to baste skin in rich, fatty moisture (oily or normal skins might as well get something cheap). But the original bottled Creme is still absolutely wonderful on my dry skin. Regular use certainly improves skin condition over time, but it's what I use occasionally when I'm going somewhere special, when I want my bodycare to hold up to a posh perfume, blow dry, make-up and frock. Because Creme de Corps is an expensive treat, albeit one that goes an awfully long way. Don't make the mistake of thinking you can get round the problem by buying cheaply from eBay. Kiehl's simple packaging (unless one of the very lovely limited edition Creme de Corps designs) is way too easy for counterfeiters to mimic and you end up with something similar to UHT milk tinted with yellow food colouring. I bear the mental scars.

Having spent my childhood coated in thick, unctuous petroleum-based lotions in a host of generic white bottles, itching like mad and being teased mercilessly by classmates, I really should hate Eucerin. It's an unsexy, slightly joyless brand that makes skincare feel like a chore not the pleasure it can be. And yet weirdly, it has slipped past my firewall against mineral oil-rich pharmacy-shelf brands, and somehow occupied a place close to my heart. There are some excellent products in the range, some of which I've been recommending for many years. The Hyaluron Filler serum and creams, for example, are brilliant on dry and dehydrated skin, plumping up lines and restoring some perk.

But Eucerin's icon comes in the form of Aquaphor, an ointment used widely since 1925 in medicine and in homes, nicknamed 'The Duct Tape of dermatology' by the very many doctors who swear by it. For them, Aquaphor's appeal lies in its 'semi-occlusive' formula, meaning that while it traps in moisture and provides a barrier against germs, it still allows oxygen and moisture to reach the skin to aid wound healing. For beauty lovers, Aquaphor offers uncommon versatility. It works as an excellent humectant on dry lips, wind-chapped limbs and cuticles, as a tamer of brows and a subtle gloss for mouth and cheeks, a curer of nappy rash, and as a handy barrier against hair dye staining (just apply it around the hairline before mixing the colourant, then leave it until you've done your final rinse). It contains mineral oil, and so I wouldn't recommend it as a face cream – although plenty happily use it as one without breakouts or irritation – but regardless of skin type, it's well worth keeping a tube in your bathroom for all else.

It's true to say that it's much harder for a small company to create an icon than it is for some huge multinational whose research, development, marketing, advertising and PR spend is, metaphorically speaking, a bottomless cup of coffee. It's perhaps harder still to do it while refusing to compromise on your principles of self-sustainability and all-natural formulas, and yet the thoroughly good eggs at Burt's Bees somehow pulled it off. It started in Maine, when local artist and single mum Roxanne Quimby was trying to thumb a ride home. Burt Shavitz, a local beekeeper who sold honey from the back of his truck, stopped. The pair got chatting and Burt offered to give Roxanne any unused wax from his hives, so she could make it into candles. The candles, fashioned into fruits and vegetables, were beautiful, and their success allowed the pair to fund their next project, a beeswax lip balm.

To say this sweet, simple, natural, homespun product took off would be to grossly understate the achievements of Burt's Bees. The cruelty-free lip balm, devoid of traditional ingredients of petroleum jelly, mineral oil or camphor, packaged in either its classic round bee print tin or a convenient stick, is a product that sums up perfectly the cult beauty movement of the 1990s, where customers sought out quirky, one-off products by cool brands outside the megabrand triumvirate of L'Oréal – Estée Lauder – LVMH. Burt's Bees' message of authenticity, nature and simplicity was, and still is, extremely appealing. I can think of no other product that infiltrated the snobbish cult beauty market via the shelves of health food stores, or as a novelty item sold in gift shops, and yet by virtue of being both effective and rather lovely, this succeeded. Burt's Bees' pluck, size and product range are already enough for me, before even factoring in what a thoroughly decent company it is. There are now many good products in the Burt's Bees range (the Almond and Milk Hand Cream, which smells intoxicatingly like newborn babies wrapped in marzipan blankets, is my favourite), but the first and bestselling lip balm formula remains its queen bee.

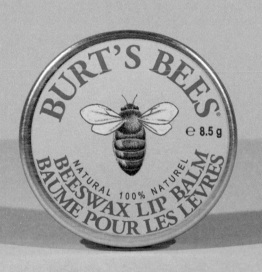

There are several reasons Advanced Night Repair deserves both your respect and its iconic status. Launched in 1982, it was the world's first consumer skincare serum. The idea behind it was that unlike moisturising creams, which have to pack in emollients, sun protection and thickening agents to deliver the right protective texture, a serum could have a much finer texture, smaller molecules and be stuffed predominantly with ingredients that fixed specific skin concerns. While a cream sat on the top of the skin, an inherently finer serum could dig a little deeper. In creating Night Repair (the 'Advanced' came later, and since then, it's been known in the business as simply 'ANR'), Estée Lauder completely changed the conversation around skincare. We were no longer talking merely about lovely creams that made us feel nice, but questioning the old wives' belief that mere moisture kept skin looking its best. ANR was about specific problem-solving with active ingredients, and when it came to choosing those ingredients, the Lauder team struck gold.

Hyaluronic acid is a viscous fluid substance found naturally in the human body, particularly around the eyes and connective tissue, where its primary function is to keep things moist, mobile and comfortable. Its magic is in its ability to hold a thousand times its weight in water. Scientists began to wonder if its topical use could help dehydrated, crêpey, ageing skin do the same, plumping it up a little, like a raisin dropped in warm water. The research team at Lauder felt it could, and combined the hyaluronic acid with antioxidants and other actives to build the world's first skin serum. The effect hyaluronic acid has had on beauty products across every price point and category cannot be overstated – it's in practically everything you'd ever want to put on your face. It's the one ingredient whose absence I will almost immediately notice. Estée Lauder Advanced Night Repair was so unique and so revolutionary that even now, when the market is rammed with serums for every conceivable purpose, it still has over twenty-five worldwide patents and patents pending, and remains one of the world's bestselling serums.

Whether or not you like ANR (and ironically, as I get older, I find its hyaluronic punch lands a bit too softly for me personally and the recent revamp – distinguished by a 'II' after its name – was fine, but something of a missed opportunity), its impact on skincare globally has been absolutely enormous. The little apothecary bottle and pipette dropper we now just accept as standard serum packaging? ANR did it first. The concept of repairing past damage with skincare? Lauder invented it with ANR. A skincare revolution in one little brown bottle, ANR is a true beauty icon without whom your bathroom shelf might now look very different indeed.

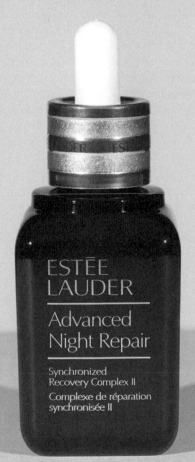

This is a perfect example of how subjective skincare can be. For a good ten years, all any dermatologist seemed to recommend was Cetaphil, a relatively inexpensive and unfussy rinse-off cleanser available widely in the States but not, at that time, in the UK. While moisturiser, mask and serum recommendations were varied, Cetaphil seemed to be the doctors' default cleanser of choice for almost any skincare gripe. If you had rosacea – try Cetaphil; if you were sensitive – stick to Cetaphil; if you'd just had a facelift – wash only in Cetaphil; if you were acne prone – well, you get it, I'm sure. The endless and uncritical love for Cetaphil was especially enticing to me because I have a serious obsession with American drugstores, and a disproportionate love for tracking down hard-to-find products. Truly, I've barely dumped my suitcase and passport in my hotel room when I'm on the sidewalk, charging towards the nearest Duane Reade or Walgreens to spend 200 unnecessary dollars on wholly unsuitable products because the font on the gaudy bottle looks pleasingly foreign. And so my love for Cetaphil seemed like a done deal.

Sadly, it failed the due diligence. While the friends for whom I brought back a bottle raved about Cetaphil, I was left wondering what all the fuss was about. First, it contains sulphates. I'm not a fan of these foaming agents in skincare, though I quite understand those who need the psychological boost of a foam. The problem is that Cetaphil is so low-foaming that one gets the worst of both worlds: my skin feels drier, only without that sense of squeaky cleanliness. Second, and for me crucially, Cetaphil is no good at all at removing make-up. The most thorough-seeming cleanse will still result in orange smears on the towel, making Cetaphil advisable only as a second night-time step. This flaw sums up my long-held belief that while dermatologists – whom I have utterly revered and valued since early childhood – are the final word on the science of skincare, their insight is often poor when it comes to real life outside a lab or surgery.

What I mean by that is while a great derm can tell you exactly which sunblock will best protect the skin without clogging pores, they will rarely know if it also peels off in lumps the minute you apply your foundation, rendering unusable even the best product in the world. Doctors are rightly thinking about skin health and efficacy, not lifestyle and quality of use. They correctly obsess over ingredients, while not always acknowledging that overall texture, packaging and formula can be the difference between addictive and useless. And so I concluded that Cetaphil was, for me, one such case in point. Almost everything about this legendary product looks good on paper, and I can understand why it's so respected by doctors, even loved by so many consumers. It just doesn't work for my life.

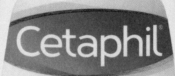

Cetaphil®

Gentle Skin Cleanser

 Face & Body Dry, sensitive skin

Non-comedogenic
Fragrance-free
Soap-free
236 ml ℮

I realised the other day when completing my online grocery shop that I buy more products by Dove than any other brand. To be fully transparent, I am extraordinarily lucky in that I don't generally pay for many products at all – everything is sent to me before launching in the hope I like it and write something favourable. What I do buy is deodorant, razor blades, handwash, bar soap, toothpaste, shower cream and body lotion, mainly because when it comes to these items specifically I'm quite uncharacteristically brand loyal and have little appetite to experiment unless a work assignment demands it. Dove caters for many of my household toiletry needs: the shower cream (especially the Silk Glow version) stands permanently in the bathroom, cap flipped and ready for action. The original deodorant is the only one, I think, that doesn't spoil the smell of a good shower with obtrusive scent. *Desert Island Discs* while soaking in Dove's almondy bath foam is one of life's true and guiltless pleasures. The liquid handwash, deliciously creamy and cheap, is the one I decant into the prettier bottles of luxury brands long since drained by my extravagant and undiscerning children.

Ironically, the one incarnation of Dove that I don't like (men's range aside, with its pointlessly gender-specific take on the already lovely unisex Dove scent) is the very foundation of every one of its products, and the only one truly deserving of the term 'icon'. The Beauty Bar, launched in 1957, is a face soap and therefore no amount of added moisturiser – famously one quarter here – can persuade me to use it anywhere above the shoulders.

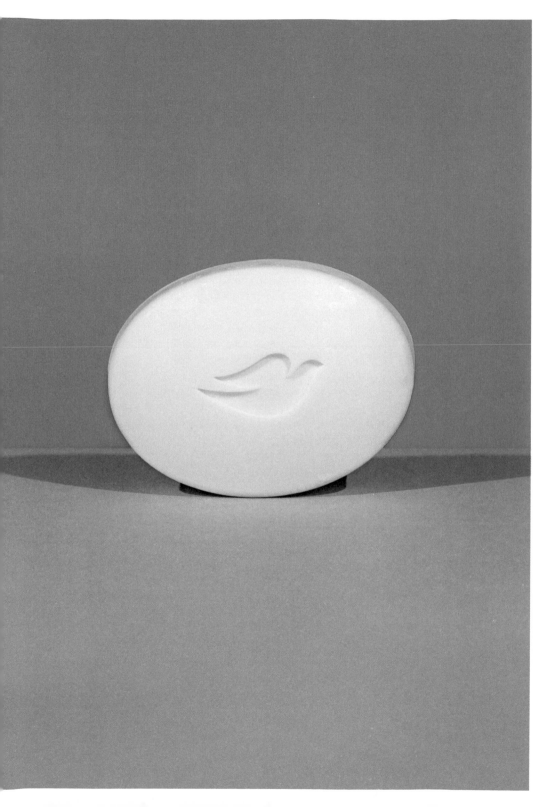

The irony with Neutrogena is that I tend to back the wrong horse. One of my favourite products of all time is its Body Emulsion, an absolute godsend for serious dry skin sufferers that they've twice tried to discontinue (at time of writing, it is available again as Deep Moisture, but I live in a mild state of fear). I almost unfailingly adore Neutrogena suncare, and yet they choose not to sell it in Europe. The wonderful, moisturising Original Rainbath shower gel has been withdrawn from general circulation and must now be obtained like some grubby porno from online importers, and as for their peerless mid-price, retinol-based, anti-ageing skincare – will they ever see fit to share the love with Britain? Meanwhile, the appeal of Neutrogena's internationally celebrated icons, namely T/Gel dandruff shampoo and Norwegian Formula Hand Cream, eludes me.

Nonetheless, one cannot deny that the stiff, rather unyielding concentrated cream based on a traditional recipe used by Norwegian fishermen on their sore, wind-chapped hands, has earned its place in beauty history. Because those who use it are evangelical about it, and I won't begin to tell them they're wrong. And yet funnily enough, the thing people love about Norwegian Formula – the ungreasy, dry-touch texture so uncommon in hand creams – is the very thing I can't bear about it. The large amount of glycerin (an excellent old ingredient, I'll readily admit) makes for a strange, slightly waxy feeling that I can't seem to ignore. It certainly moisturises well, if temporarily, and I love the soft, comforting smell of the original, fragranced, version. But apart from that, Norwegian Formula Hand Cream just doesn't float my sea trawler. In my typical fashion, however, I do really love the less popular Norwegian Formula Fast Absorbing Hand Cream, though I'm afraid the mere act of my putting that in writing may jinx its very existence.

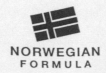

NORWEGIAN
FORMULA

hand
cream

CONCENTRATED

instant relief of dry, chapped hands
just a dab needed

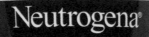

Neutrogena®

DERMATOLOGIST TESTED

Oh Sisley, with your aloof, impenetrable French packaging, unknowable department store counters and your bonkers price points, so inaccessible to the vast majority of beauty lovers. I wish you weren't so damn lovely. This is the mask used by supermodels after six straight weeks of sleepless, over-made-up, skin-terrorising service. It's the mask reserved by make-up artists for only the best magazine covers and gold-band clientele. It's the mask I give to women at their lowest ebb, when divorce, bereavement or illness has ravaged the body, mind and soul. Rich, luxurious, gentle and soothing, a ten-minute session with Black Rose Cream Mask is like your most well-off girlfriend taking you for a four-hour lunch and three bottles from the lower half of the wine list.

MASQUE CREME
A LA ROSE NOIRE
Instant Jeunesse
Lisse, repulpe, illumine

BLACK ROSE
CREAM MASK
Instant Youth
Smoothing, plumping,
brightening

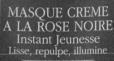

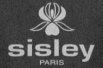

sisley
PARIS

NET WT. 2.1 OZ.   61 g 60 ml

When I first moved to London, aged 15, Molton Brown was the coolest hair salon around. Opened in 1973 and named after its home, South Molton Street, and Brown's fashion store, located a few doors down and owned by Molton Brown's founder Caroline Burstein's parents, Molton Brown was where Sam McKnight – arguably the most successful session hairstylist of all time – made his name, and was among the first of a teenage Kate Moss's modelling clients.

Molton Brown specialised in natural hairstyling techniques at a time when harsh chemical treatments and heated tools were all the rage, and their sought-after product was the 'Molton Browner', a dusty-pink quilted bendy roller, stiffened with a wire loop, that was wound into sections of hair and slept in overnight. I was gifted a dozen by my Aunt Sue and though I was wholly inept at using them (the resulting style was reliably disastrous), they were so pretty, so unlike anything I'd ever seen, that I adored them out of all proportion.

I finally got to visit the salon myself when they opened a little shop in reception. Here, they sold body lotions and soaps, and unexpectedly pro-grade beauty kit. It was here I bought my first ever make-up brush roll (I still have it) and my first bottle of Orange & Bergamot Hand Wash. I would never have believed that this ancillary product in a line known for its haircare would become a beauty phenomenon, launch an entire category of luxury handwashes (paving the way for wonderful brands like Cowshed and L'Occitane) and be copied so mercilessly worldwide. Nowadays, handwash and hand cream are the products for which Molton Brown is best known. They are the sign of a good-quality boutique hotel, an unfailingly well-received token of love on Mother's Day, and a clear message of gratitude to a teacher at the end of term. Their high-quality natural oils make for delicate, authentic scents and gentle, skin-softening cleansing.

Sadly, the same cannot be said for the dozens of brands and retailers who've exploited Molton Brown's cachet and very modest, easily replicated packaging, and knocked up their own. I'm all for a designer dupe, whether a Miu Miu-inspired coat from Topshop or an Eames-style desk bought in IKEA, but there's no doubt that over the years Molton Brown has seen its excellent product devalued by impostors. Worse still is the common practice of businesses refilling real Molton Brown bottles with some industrial soap bought in Costco, sending an illusory message of luxury. I can't imagine how many people assume they're using the real thing then wonder, as they breathe in the smell of car air freshener, what all the fuss is about.

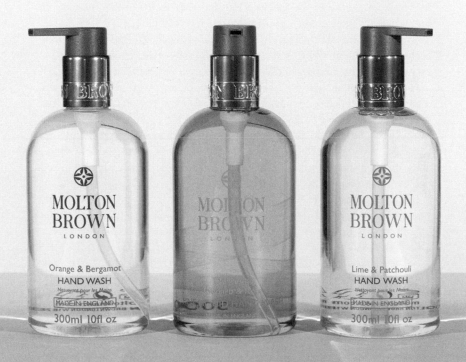

Some time around my seventh or eighth birthday, my mother returned home from Cardiff with a bottle of Cocoa Butter Hand & Body Lotion from one of the very first branches of Body Shop. She'd engaged the sales consultant in conversation, told her about my dry, scaly, inherited skin condition, and been promised that cocoa butter would help. The lotion was nothing short of revelatory and marked a huge turning point in my life. I'd previously used only horrible, NHS-prescribed bath oils and emollient creams that sat thickly on the surface of my skin, smelling like hospitals and never sinking into anything other than my school tights. Conversely, the Body Shop lotion sank a little better into my skin, soothing, softening and making it smell of Milky Bar chocolate. That one bottle of lotion set me down a path of skincare obsession. I began tweaking the cocoa butter – adding olive oil from the kitchen, pouring it into baths, mixing it with Tate & Lyle to slough off the flakes before a soak. The only problem with the Body Shop lotion was that it did leave an oleaginous film on my skin, and didn't improve its overall tone and evenness (I looked a bit pink and veiny) and so I began searching for an alternative.

I found Palmer's Cocoa Butter Formula Lotion on an Afro-Caribbean beauty stall while skiving off school in an indoor market and soon found my prayers answered. This – the world's bestselling cocoa butter product – sinks in more rapidly and thoroughly than any other I've found, smooths skin, banishes the occasional ashiness of brown and black skins and leaves all legs with an even, healthier-looking tone. It softens limbs, cuticles, elbows, feet, scalp and babies' bums, and smells of holidays, warm beaches and of ice-cream sundaes melting in hot chocolate sauce. Its cheerfully cheap price tag means it can be treated like an essential family household item and slathered on with abandon whenever dryness strikes. There are now dozens of products in the Palmer's range, but the true icon here is the waxy formulation sold in tubs (don't be put off by its solidity: the secret to cocoa butter's success is that it's the only known natural moisturiser that melts at body temperature).

That said, I now much more often use Palmer's anti-ageing cocoa butter with added exfoliating alpha and beta hydroxy acids, which stinks to high heaven, but sloughs my skin brilliantly when it's going through its twice-yearly seasonal transition meltdown. It works better than anything I've tried at any price and as a not entirely welcome bonus, works as an excellent insect repellent and chastening contraceptive.

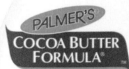

I can think of few make-up items more celebrated than this. So numerous are its awards, so uncritical is its feedback, so enduring is its appeal that two decades after its 1996 launch, Laura Mercier's Tinted Moisturizer is starting to look like the smug class swot. The problem is that one must grudgingly concede that it really still is the best. Because unlike most other brands, what Laura Mercier – a make-up artist who's always been far more interested in the complexion than in colour – realised is that even though most of us want a sheer, effortless, healthy-looking base for casual days, we still want *something*. Her response was to create the make-up equivalent of a 10-denier stocking – evening out blotches, masking imperfections, all the while pretending to represent what God gave us.

It proved so successful that two variations soon joined it. The Classic Tinted Moisturizer formula has good light reflection and remains the best and most flattering for most people. But I also love the illuminating version which, while a tad too shimmery and space-age for some tastes, mixes beautifully with practically any other complexion make-up to add a subtler glow. The oil-free edition is perfect for combination, oily or skins losing their usual make-up to regular hot flashes. All three versions include a decent enough SPF20 for autumn and winter use, come in racially inclusive shades with a flattering neutral or yellow undertone, and blend like a dream over day cream or primer (I wouldn't actually advise anyone to use any tint as their main skincare, though I've been known to apply this straight over facial sunblock in summer).

In Tinted Moisturizer, Mercier unwittingly created the reference point for all others and has raised the bar across the industry. Tinted moisturisers have evolved and improved considerably to snatch a share of the market, while BB and CC creams have tried to make the entire category look outmoded and déclassé. But none has managed to offer both the coverage and glow of Laura's original – still among my all-time top five favourite bases.

laura mercier

TINTED MOISTURIZER SPF 20 ● BASE HYDRATANTE TEINTÉE IP 20
NUDE

Smells that will always remind me of summer: cut grass, new flip-flops on warm tarmac, a sunbathing dog's belly, hot car, a fresh jug of Pimm's, melted chocolate, fragrant basil on the windowsill, sausages on a barbecue and Hawaiian Tropic sun lotion on my arms. One whiff of this sticky, sexy, sunny coconutty smell and I'm transported instantly to my first parent-free holiday abroad, lying on the beach reading *Sky* magazine and listening to George Michael's *Listen Without Prejudice Vol. I*, smoking duty-free menthols, sipping too-sweet vodka punch and gossiping with girlfriends about boys in desperate need of offloading. Sadly, like most Hawaiian Tropic users in the 1990s, I was woefully under protected. Factor 8 oil was as precautionary as it got – we were still fostering the deluded belief that we might turn the colour of J.Lo and not be picking peeled skin off our shins in a month's time.

I can't claim to use Hawaiian Tropic all that often these days, though I still have quite the weakness for their delicious Coconut Body Butter (as cheap as chips and available everywhere). For sun protection, I'm more likely to pack Clinique, Nivea or Clarins. But I love to have a brown spray bottle of the original Hawaiian Tropic oil in the bathroom, if only to wear as an occasional fragrance, spritzing it on my skin to instantly lift my mood. Because Hawaiian Tropic suntan oil is the bottled smell of long, happy summers.

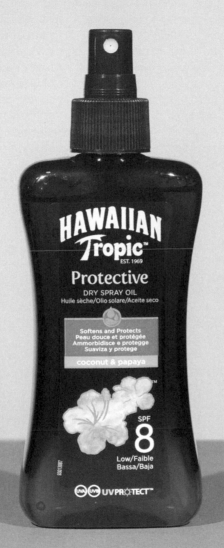

Now pushing 60, Elnett is approaching the age of the women I associated it with – and aspired to be – when I was a child. To me, it's old-school, well-groomed, posh-nan-in-a-can.

In fact Elnett, satisfyingly sold in the same immediately recognisable brushed gold canisters since 1962 (with the line-drawn woman's face added two years later), is good enough to find currency with every age group.

More expensive than many other sprays, it doesn't offer the strongest hold available – you might choose something else for a beehive or serious backcombing. But it justifies the outlay with one invaluable characteristic: you can brush it out and start again. Elnett was the first hairspray to oblige in this way, thanks to the inclusion of fine polymers in its formula. Previous hair lacquers, missing the magic ingredient, had been rather gluey and unmanageable. If you messed up your 'do, you were quite literally stuck. Elnett keeps hair mobile, waves bouncy and you don't hit the town feeling like you're sporting a coiff fashioned from teak by a master carpenter. Thanks to its static-preventing properties, it even stops dresses sticking to (sprayed) tights. But Elnett might never have seen the light of day had it not been for the persistence of L'Oréal head François Dalle, who had seen an initial incarnation of the product fail to find favour in salons. Undeterred, he had the spray repackaged, renamed (initially) 'Ellenet' and successfully market-tested before becoming a huge success in both salons and shops.

Until 2010, Elnett (effectively French for 'she neat') was unavailable in the USA, obliging top American session hairstylists to stock up in Europe and squirrel it back home for use on cover shoots and catwalk shows. The effort and extra luggage fees required to score some Elnett added hugely to its cult status and desirability, and gradually Elnett became known as the fashion industry's lacquer of choice. Elnett's star remains undimmed – even now, two cans are sold in Britain every five seconds. It comes in a variety of formulas but each offers that distinctive, deliciously chemical, Elnett aroma. It's the smell I associate closely with the ritual of getting ready with girlfriends – Diana Ross on the Sonos, glass of Prosecco on the go, hovering hands shielding the bubbles against falling Elnett. It's the smell of a night out and of good times ahead.

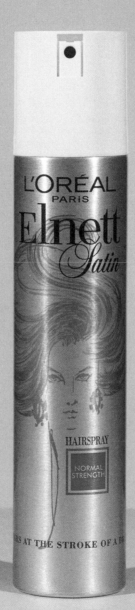

One of the great sadnesses of my career is that I never worked with Kevyn Aucoin. Along with Mary Greenwell and François Nars, this extraordinarily talented, decent and visionary make-up artist was responsible for the looks that inspired my deep love of beauty and, consequently, my future career. I still read his books, search YouTube for the many catwalk shows he worked on, and see his vast influence on so many of today's beauty looks (you know the heavily contoured, sharp-browed, nude-toned faces you see everywhere on Instagram in 2016? Kevyn Aucoin invented them way before Kim Kardashian reached for her first Beautyblender. And he did it with uncommon elegance and finesse). But more on that later. It's our great fortune that two years prior to his death, Aucoin put his expertise into his own make-up line, having spent years creating products for Revlon and Shiseido.

In industry terms, a number of Aucoin's original and endlessly copied products could fairly be classed as iconic. Celestial Powder, a golden highlighter, was devised after Aucoin went in to say goodnight to his niece and found her sleepy face bathed in the beautiful glow of her bedroom nightlight. He wanted a product to cheat the effect and to this day Celestial Powder comes closer than anything else. His two mascaras – curling and thickening – were the first Western takes on Asian tubing formulations, and allowed me, and many others, to be smudge-free for the first time.

But I think the most special and groundbreaking product in the Kevyn Aucoin line is Sensual Skin Enhancer. This extraordinarily thick paste is ostensibly a foundation, but it's an unhelpful categorisation that would scare many customers away. What Sensual Skin Enhancer really is, is a multi-purpose skin-toned pigment cream. On first sight it looks too unyielding to blend over the face, but in this untouched state Sensual Skin Enhancer is actually a full coverage concealer so opaque that it can cover tattoos, scars and birthmarks in just a few pats of the fingertip. To completely cover a spot, press the tiniest dot over the redness. To make a glowing, dewy, skin-tone unifying foundation, mix a rice grain-sized amount of Sensual Skin Enhancer with a blob of illuminator or primer. For a healthy-looking tinted moisturiser, just mix with day cream. For highlighter, choose a paler shade; for contouring, a darker one. It is sweat-proof, rainproof, racially inclusive, non-glaring and long-wearing (expect twenty hours of even coverage. Yes, really), making it a perfect choice for brides. One tiny jar should last you about a year. Aucoin's influence on beauty will last for ever.

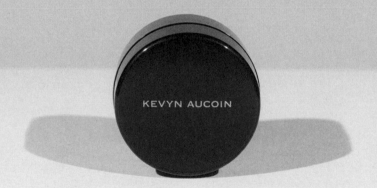

THE
NOSTALGICS

Cold cream is one of those products you feel surprised still exists. It seems like the kind of thing seen only on the backstage dressing tables of vintage ballerinas or vaudeville performers, for the purpose of removing heavy pancake foundation and character make-up. And yet you can still find cold cream – usually Pond's – in practically any chemist. Part of me wants to bob behind the shelf to see whether anyone under 90 is buying it. Instead, I recently satisfied my curiosity by buying some for myself and giving it a go for possibly only the second time in my life. It's a thick, unctuous white cream, made mainly of mineral oil (which my dry skin generally doesn't mind – I wouldn't be so experimental if I was oily and more spot-prone) that's massaged into the face to dissolve make-up, before being wiped off with cotton wool, tissues or a wet flannel. And here's the thing: it works brilliantly within that limited brief. Like any heavy emollient, it left my face feeling soft, and removed make-up clean away – including heavy mascara. It was remarkably gentle, even when smeared carelessly over my eyes.

Pond's is the true icon among cold creams, on account of its age (launched in 1914, it was based on a patented medicine, Golden Treasure, invented by New York pharmacist Theron T. Pond way back in 1846 and became an instant hit with society ladies and showbiz performers), classic tub (I've never owned it until now and yet I'd always recognise it from twenty paces – quite an achievement), its influence on beauty generally (Pond's deserves huge credit for pioneering the use of exfoliating AHAs in mass-market beauty products) and the propensity of some female celebrities to deny dieting, litres of Botox and plastic surgery and insist their raving beauty is down to 'burgers, good genes and a dot of Pond's Cold Cream'. It's become a hilarious celebrity shorthand for 'I'm so casual about my looks' that, while utterly disingenuous nonsense, has rather added to the product's romance and mystique. I'm keeping it on my shelf for now.

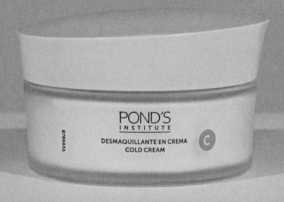

This face powder may be the most influential product you've never heard of. In 1881 most women were wearing lead-based, heavily perfumed face powders to achieve the pale, matte look of the day. Concerned that women were literally poisoning themselves in the name of beauty, renowned cosmetic pharmacist Théophile LeClerc went to his basement and created an extremely light-textured alternative by grinding up zinc oxide, rice starch, coloured pigment and a smidge of talc. He made six different shades, one of them Banane, a soft, flattering yellow to add radiance. One hundred and nine years later, I bought my first tin of Banane powder in a professional supply store on the request of my boss, the make-up artist Lynne Easton. Every professional used yellow loose powder back then, either alone to brighten, or mixed in with skin shades to give them a more flattering undertone, long before department store brands had got the memo. T. LeClerc, Leichner and Kryolan were used most commonly, but I think the first is most deserving of the term 'icon'.

It remains a cult favourite today, reinvigorated by the trend for colour correction (there are pink, lilac, apricot and green versions of the original powder, as well as a number of skin tones), the unstoppable shift towards contouring and the insatiable interest in professional make-up artistry and supplies. It helps, of course, that the embossed metallic T. LeClerc pot, with its raised Belle Époque lettering like something from a vintage absinthe bottle, is such a thing of rare beauty. It elevates it from good powder to something very special, that deserves to be applied with a marabou feather puff by someone in a blush satin nightie and finger waves.

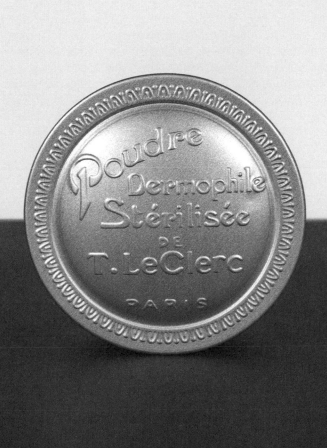

I think, to be entirely honest, that American readers could make a very strong case for naming the original Skin Cream (now called Original Deep Cleansing Cream) as Noxzema's beauty icon. Developed in 1914 as a sunburn remedy, this mentholated ointment was quickly appropriated for the removal of make-up and the cleaning of chapped and irritated skin. Much as I love the heritage of Noxzema skin cream, I can't personally claim to be a fan (it's a bit like cleansing with Carmex lip balm). But what do hold notional, practical and iconic appeal for me are Noxzema's excellent shaving foams. These colour-coded tins of dense, rich, creamy foam pride themselves on their suitability for dry, sensitive or acne-prone skins often aggravated by others.

I myself am a great lover of the Cocoa Butter variety for leg shaving purposes, but I'd be lying if I claimed the packaging was not a contributing factor. Noxzema tins, with their simple fonts, generic primary colours and satisfyingly chubby stature are, I think, remarkably beautiful and evocative of a simpler, more wholesome time. They have the kind of packaging that could be identified as 1950s American from a mile away, without your quite being able to explain why. One imagines reductive scenes involving dads standing at a basin, shaving for another day's work, driving door to door in a Cadillac to sell aluminium siding to suburban housewives. On a shelf with Euthymol toothpaste and Black & White hair wax, Noxzema foams become way more than mere toiletries, they are an interior design classic in themselves. And for just a little over a fiver.

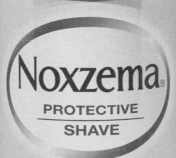

Noxzema®
PROTECTIVE
SHAVE

SHAVING FOAM
Cocoa Butter

Conditioning

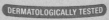
DERMATOLOGICALLY TESTED

300 ml e

I feel neither shame nor embarrassment when I say I absolutely love this perfume. I think it was my mother – a woman of good taste and zero snobbery – who first introduced me to it when I was a little girl during its 1970s heyday (though it's been around since 1927). For many, L'Aimant is as evocative of that time as the smell of Babycham and Black Forest gateau, furniture polish and warm shagpile carpets. But to dismiss it as retro is to miss out on what remains a very lovely scent. Created by the great François Coty, L'Aimant is a warm, comforting aldehydic floral that's not too sweet or overpowering. It's absolutely bargainous, of course, and yet it still smells like a woman of means and elegance. I love its quiet, unpretentious confidence. If you like Chanel No 5, you will probably like this. And even if you don't, it's only a tenner. Try it anyway.

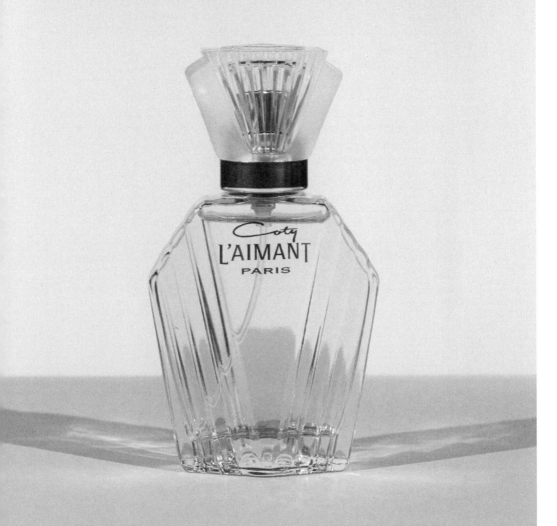

No official figures are available but I'd be prepared to bet almost any sum on Anaïs Anaïs having been the most popular perfume among teens of the 1980s, and very possibly beyond. Launched in 1978, Anaïs Anaïs was like the beautiful new girl everyone wanted to show around school. The dreamy Sarah Moon-photographed advertising campaign, the gorgeous and pleasingly bulbous white opaque glass bottle, the scent of airy white flowers and soft, cuddly basenotes of amber and sandalwood made for a pretty intoxicating cocktail for the average teenage girl more used to cider and black. It was almost everyone's first proper perfume (Benetton Colors came later) and certainly the first to make teenagers feel it was for them, not their mums.

Personally, I never wore Anaïs Anaïs. It seemed, from my perspective, to be a perfume for swots. It was worn by straight-A sixth formers with perfect demi-waves, carrying indexed ring binders and exercise books carefully jacketed in brown paper. It was too genteel, too prim, too safe for an indie girl with a Madonna duvet cover. I was magnetically drawn to Loulou, Anaïs Anaïs's almost tear-jerkingly potent little sister. Loulou was (and still is) the scent of ripe fruit, sticky vanilla and big, white and yellow flowers on the pull. It's the Rizzo to Anaïs's Sandy – not demure, polite or tasteful, but hot, bold and bags of fun. It has spirit, even if a bit too much for comfort. Mine came in an opaque, turquoise, faceted glass atomiser trimmed in merlot (the original was a beautifully bonkers art nouveau bowl and stopper) and I still, some thirty years later, believe it to be one of the loveliest perfume bottles of all time (if you love the Miu Miu perfume bottle, you'll appreciate this). If Anaïs Anaïs was for good girls, then Loulou was for bad girls. Both remain true beauty icons and brilliant, important scents. But there was never really a chance of my going any other way.

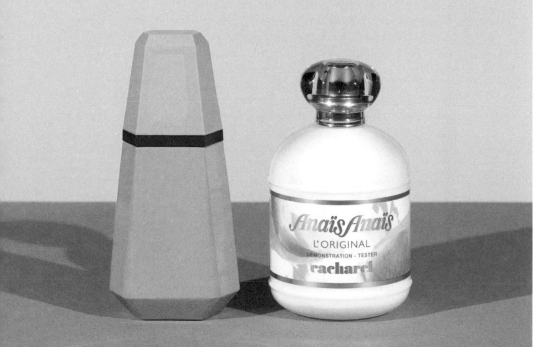

I've never before tracked down a product after hearing about it in a song, but that's exactly what happened when, at the age of 11, I became obsessed with *Transformer*, the 1972 album by Lou Reed. Everyone, I think, has a record that first alerts them to a world outside chart music and the family's existing collection, and feels extremely, and enduringly, personal to them. For me, *Transformer* was that album and track six, 'Make Up', seemed like a particularly significant joining of two of my greatest passions. In the song, a bemused and beguiled Reed observes a female partner's morning beauty routine, listing her techniques and products like lip gloss, rosehips and pan-cake. I had no idea what the last two even were, and was determined to find out. Though Reed wasn't specific about brand, it seems fitting that a song entitled 'Make Up' led me to Max Factor, the man who'd invented the term.

Max Factor's Pan-Cake was a solid, full-coverage base, developed in 1935, almost twenty years after Mr Factor had introduced the radical concept of matching complexion products to natural skin tones. The initiative was arguably the most influential in the history of make-up, and mapped the course for practically every foundation, concealer and powder thereafter, including Pan-Cake. As with so many Max Factor products, this new formula was created purely with Hollywood in mind. The development of Technicolor film meant that any surrounding colours were reflected onto the slightly shiny greasepaint on the faces of starlets. The effect was so unflattering that many stars refused to appear in colour at all.

It was Max Factor's son Frank who found the solution in this rather heavy yet flexible, transfer-resistant, matte, skin-coloured cream to be applied with a damp sponge to cover any flaws for many hours at a time. It debuted in the film *Vogues of 1938* (1937), followed by *The Goldwyn Follies* a few months later, and soon Pan-Cake became the standard for all Technicolor filmmaking. Consequently, public demand for Pan-Cake was so huge that Max Factor developed new, lighter shades for consumer use away from the glare of strong studio lighting. It immediately became the fastest and largest selling single make-up item to date, and easily one of the most revolutionary beauty products of all time.

For new glamour TODAY—
a young-looking skin TOMORROW!

WHEN you make up, think of tomorrow as well as today...choose "Pan-Cake", the original, which because of its exclusive patented formula does two things...it creates glamour for today and safeguards the skin against sun and wind which may bring drying, harshening, aging signs tomorrow. Once you try "Pan-Cake", you'll be devoted to it forever *because...*

★ *It creates a lovely new complexion; there's a color harmony shade for your type*

★ *It gives the skin a softer, smoother, younger look; the formula guards against drying*

★ *It takes just a few seconds to make up; and stays on for hours without re-touching*

★ *It helps hide tiny complexion faults; your make-up always looks fresh and lovely*

And remember, there's only one "Pan-Cake", the original, created by *Max Factor Hollywood* Tested and proved perfect by famous screen stars and millions of lovely girls and women everywhere. Make up with Pan-Cake today for your most thrilling adventure in new beauty.

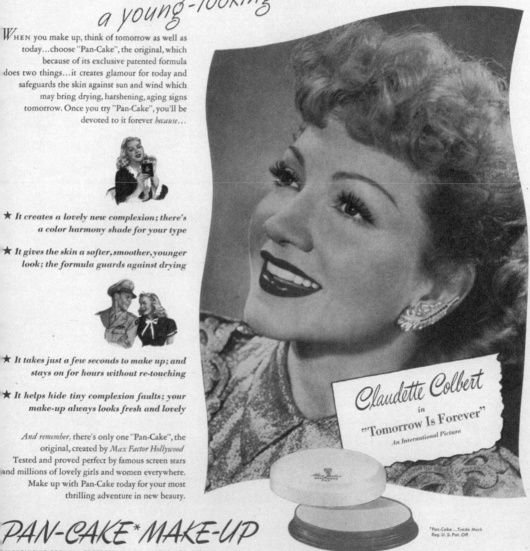

Claudette Colbert
in
"Tomorrow Is Forever"
An International Picture

PAN-CAKE * MAKE-UP

AN EXCLUSIVE FORMULA PROTECTED BY U.S. PATENT NOS. 2034697-2101834

*Pan-Cake ...Trade Mark Reg. U.S. Pat. Off.

ORIGINATED BY MAX FACTOR HOLLYWOOD

I think I can honestly say that in each of the years of my teens and twenties, I felt Oil of Ulay Beauty Fluid on my skin. It was the kind of moisturiser you would reliably find on the bathroom shelf wherever you went, whether home with a school friend for a nightie party or, later, with a man for a different variety of sleepover. As long as there was Oil of Ulay, you needed nothing beyond a toothbrush to feel sufficiently equipped.

Oil of Ulay (Olay in the US) was launched in 1952 as a lighter alternative to the rich, thick, oily creams of the day. This thin, milky moisturiser (created by chemist Graham Wulff and containing glycerin, lanolin and mineral oils) would sink straight into the face and neck without rubbing or greasiness and in this regard was way ahead of its time. Also unusual was how Olay was marketed. Wulff took out a heap of advertising in the *Reader's Digest*, explaining very little about the product (even the name Beauty Fluid gave nothing away about what the product actually did) and waited for women to be sufficiently intrigued that they'd ask their chemist where they might find some. Orders piled up and a phenomenon was born.

In 1999 new owners Procter & Gamble decided to change the UK and Ireland brand name of Oil of Ulay to Olay, to fall in line with the American market, and set about making huge changes to the cosy nana brand it had become. And certainly, under its new name, Olay has gone on to become one of the world's leading skincare brands, and, along with Nivea, has invented an entire category of 'Masstige' (mass-market prestige) beauty products. I frequently recommend Olay Regenerist serums and creams on the basis that when budget is a consideration, it's worth investing in brands with an unlimited one, who have the very best in research and development to pass on to you. But I'm just as impressed that in among the neopeptides, niacinamide, acids and vitamin complexes, stands a simple, glycerin-based, soft pink 'beauty fluid' that promises nothing more than moisturised skin, minus the grease. And I still say Oil of Ulay, at least when it comes to Beauty Fluid, just as I call a Snickers a Marathon, and Veet, Immac. I just don't hold with change.

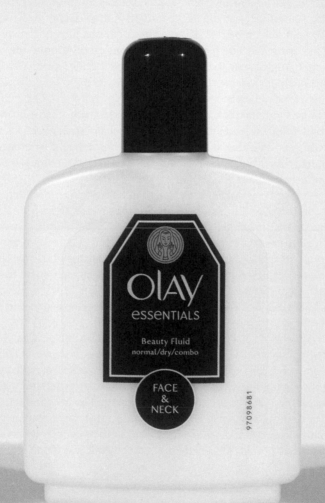

Each year, when fewer and fewer of our veterans gather at the Cenotaph, the sight of the stoic, dignified remainder becomes almost unbearably moving. As their numbers dwindle, much is being lost with them. Servicemen's societies close, memories and stories disappear, but so also do many of the quotidian habits and ephemera of that generation.

When I think of Brylcreem, I think of these veterans, impeccably turned out, preserving as best they can the habits formed in their days of active service. Originally sold only in barber's shops, Brylcreem was ideal for maintaining a smart, incorruptible side parting, an attractive proposition to any stylish 1930s gent, but invaluable in the military; in the Second World War image-conscious RAF personnel were known as the Brylcreem Boys. With the canny recruitment for its advertising campaigns of Denis Compton – one of Britain's most popular sportsmen of the era, a man so blessed with athletic prowess he played cricket for England and football for Arsenal – Brylcreem was woven into the zeitgeist on either side of the war. The 1950s might have proved its undoing, had the advent of the quiff with its associated structural hazards not prolonged the brand's appeal.

The 1960s, however, ushered in changes in hairstyling that rendered such uncompromising hair creams redundant. Shaggier, looser styles from Beatlesy mop-tops to long, unkempt hippy hair had no truck with Brylcreem and the brand declined until the eighties, when a 1950s revival – inspired principally by Levi's 501s, *Stand By Me* and a slightly nightmarish claymation Jackie Wilson – saw a new generation of quiff-bearers rediscover the cream's qualities. Then, some half a century after Compton's endorsement, Brylcreem embraced the nineties by signing up David Beckham, ensuring the cream would sell into the new millennium.

But Brylcreem's cachet lies with its heritage. You can still get it in the same lovely red packaging it's been in since the 1960s, but it evokes a still more distant time and calls to mind images of smartly turned out young men, smiling out of charmingly guileless black and white adverts, blissfully unaware of an oncoming war; of boisterous boys, intoxicated by beer and happiness, twirling laughing girls at noisy VE Day parties; of those wonderful men at the Cenotaph, who decades ago risked their lives for their country without a hair out of place, and proudly present themselves the same way today.

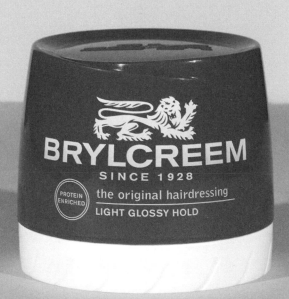

One of the most memorable scents of my childhood. We didn't always have VO5 – more often, we had the cheaper, generic apple shampoo bought in the sort of huge plastic bottles that normally contained screen wash or turps. But in either case, the shampoo inside had a strong, crisp, artificial green apple scent that was so delicious, it genuinely made your mouth water. It reminds me of Sunday nights, washing my hair in the bathwater because the rubber shower hose leapt constantly off the tap, my nightie warming on a radiator, Heinz tomato soup on the stove. It's the smell of my slightly damp pillowcase as I lay listening to Enid Blyton's *Toyland Tales*. It's the smell of Monday morning classroom. It became very hard to find in my adulthood and for years I searched for an alternative, but buying some posh organic version from Ocado seemed to be a less satisfying cheat on the real thing. Like crisps, toasters, custard creams, tinsel on a Christmas tree and bread around a bacon sandwich, apple shampoo is infinitely superior when cheap and cheerful.

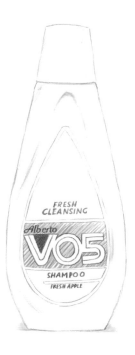

So well established are they as shorthand for a gauche, seventies notion of masculinity, it's hard to imagine that, even in their pomp, Brut and Denim could ever have been taken seriously. But maybe that's because, well, they weren't. At least not entirely.

Though we may strongly associate it with the decade of the Goodies, the kipper tie and the three-day week, it may be quite a surprise to learn that Brut actually predates The Beatles' 'Ticket to Ride'. Its seventies ubiquity is at least in part down to the launch of a budget version of Fabergé's original, containing just 33 per cent of its fragrance and accordingly named Brut 33. The deployment of British boxing icon Henry Cooper alongside a parade of high-profile sports stars including Kevin Keegan, Barry Sheene and Harvey Smith cemented Brut in the British psyche as the splash-on of choice for the cheeky-pint-before-training jack-the-lad, and Cooper's exhortation to 'splash it all over' backed up the notion that Brut 33 was accessible, non-poncey and certainly no exclusive nectar to be teased out drop by drop. Even the bottle wore a medallion.

But while Brut's geezery wink averted any danger of a descent into po-faced masculine posturing, Denim went the full testosterone mile. Hitting the market when original Brut was already nearly a teen, Denim's ad campaigns memorably featured an otherwise unseen woman's bright red nails snaking between the buttons of her feller's shirt (rendered of course in the eponymous fabric), while Bill Mitchell, high priest of the subsonic voiceover, rumbled that the fragrance was for 'the man who doesn't have to try too hard'. The chap in the ad certainly wasn't trying too hard; he was basically static for the duration, except to suddenly clamp the woman's hand when he'd seemingly had enough of – to quote another commercial of the period – her fingers doing the walking. The implication, predating by many years a similar selling proposition from Lynx, was that one splash of Denim and you'd be fighting them off with a shitty stick.

But here, perhaps, any intended tongue-in-cheek note was lost on an audience hoping Denim (the key scent element of which, perhaps counter-intuitively, was leather) might prove to be some kind of magic pulling bullet. And so it was that rather than being bought by the men who didn't have to try too hard, Denim most likely sold in greater numbers to nebbishy sales reps from Barnsley called Clive who, despite the enchanting power of their aftershave, probably had to try very hard indeed.

It's one of the most cheering stories, not just in the business of perfume, but in the history of entrepreneurship full stop. In the early 1950s Estée Lauder, then in her forties, was running a small cosmetics business with her husband Joseph. She had created her first fragrance but was struggling to position it in leading department stores, where popular perfumes were usually a brand extension for grand fashion houses and, ideally, created in France. In New York's Saks Fifth Avenue (though some accounts say this happened at Galeries Lafayette in Paris), the estimable Mrs Lauder 'accidentally' smashed a bottle of her fragrance on the floor of the perfume department, diffusing the scent and drawing enchanted women from all over the store to ask what it was they could smell. What it was they could smell was Youth-Dew, a sweet, spicy warm perfume, like a Coca-Cola reduction. It's a weighty, incensey concoction, tarry and medicinal (it features tolu balsam, used in cough syrup), but with deep amber and patchouli in its murky depths. By closing time, Lauder had been offered the space she wanted in the department. One of the ballsiest ever examples of direct marketing had paid off – and would continue to do so handsomely.

Lauder, the daughter of Jewish immigrants, was no closeted aesthete, but a brilliant, hard-selling businesswoman. She ensured that Youth-Dew's bottle cap was not sealed, so that a woman might more easily unscrew it and sniff while shopping, leaving traces of the scent on her hands in the process. She made sure samples found their way into the handbags of as many women as possible, from Princess Grace down. She encouraged retailers to include blotters impregnated with the fragrance in account customers' monthly statements. She sprayed it in the lifts of department stores. 'If I believe in something, I sell it,' she said, 'and I sell it hard.' And she had to sell hard, because Youth-Dew was launched into a market with a contradiction at its heart: a product exclusively for women, bought almost exclusively by men. In 1953 it still wasn't the done thing for a lady to buy herself a perfume. She would wait to be gifted one by her husband. And so Mrs Lauder cannily sold Youth-Dew through the back door, by ingeniously marketing it as a bath oil – something women were at liberty to buy for themselves – which could double as a perfume.

By making Youth-Dew widely affordable – it launched at $5 a bottle – Lauder now encouraged women to see fragrances in a whole new way, as something they could lavish on themselves daily, rather than reserve for special occasions. It worked: Youth-Dew sold 50,000 bottles in its first year. Mrs Lauder's resulting empire, Estée Lauder Companies, now owns a substantial number of the world's most popular beauty brands, including Clinique, Smashbox, Aveda, Bobbi Brown and Origins. Though Mrs Lauder died in 2004, her work ethic, guile and sheer moxie is indelibly marked on the business of beauty.

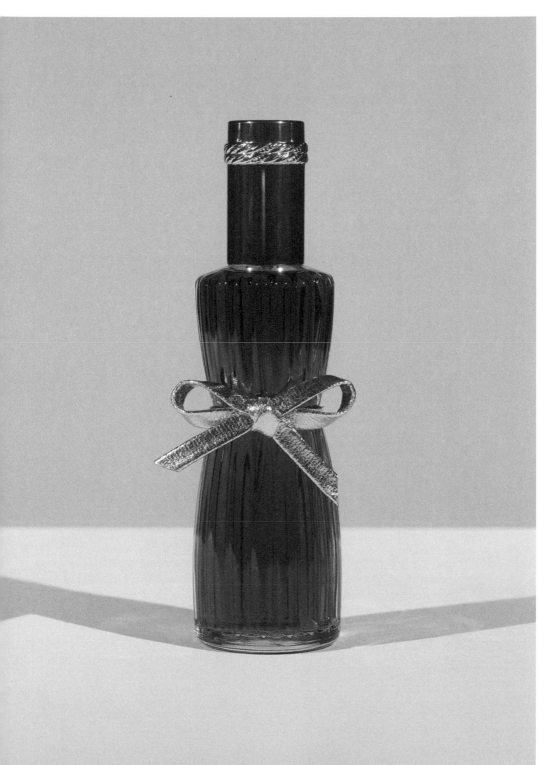

The term 'best kept secret' is applied fairly indiscriminately in the beauty press, but Frownies is one of the few products at which it can fairly be levelled. These slightly arcane and hilariously low-tech self-adhesive, anti-ageing patches are essentially Band-Aids for the face, designed to sort of stick down smoothed wrinkles and gradually train muscles not to pucker up. They definitely work, provided you're prepared to sign up for the long haul (maybe a month or so of bedtime wear for a noticeable improvement, then less frequently for top-ups). In 1889, when Elizabeth Arden was still in primary school, and way before Estée Lauder was even born, Mrs Margaret Kroesen became an unlikely beauty entrepreneur when she invented 'wrinkle eradicators' for her concert pianist daughter's 'unsightly frown lines' (okay, bit creepy, but stay with me). Impressed with the results, Kroesen put the sticky patches into production, created the B&P Company (Beauty and Personality) and sold them to Hollywood make-up designers and Broadway actors.

Show business has always used adhesives to tauten the skin (Joan Crawford, Bette Davis and Marlene Dietrich all lifted their faces with tape and secured the ends under their wigs, both off and on camera), and so Frownies proved hugely popular on set and soon became a make-up trailer staple. A Frownies patch appears on the forehead of a desperate Meryl Streep in cult classic *Death Becomes Her,* and on Glenn Close's First Lady in *Mars Attacks.* Most memorably of all, Gloria Swanson's Norma Desmond wore Frownies to bed in a desperate attempt to stave off the ageing process and preserve her Hollywood career in *Sunset Boulevard.*

But using glue and tape to smooth wrinkles is surprisingly prevalent, still. Many modern celebrities – male and female – insist on tape to lift and fix jowls and wattles (one well-known make-up artist told me of the time a former supermodel, while getting ready for a chat show, asked him to tape her as tightly as he could without curtailing her ability to speak). Frownies (dirt cheap, compared to Botox) may be a more preventative and less extreme measure, but I still know of several huge stars who insist on them (Raquel Welch and Marie Helvin gladly own up, many more won't). And although I understand why this obsession with concealing the ageing process is somewhat depressing to some (and I really do broadly agree), the beauty nerd and romantic in me can't help feeling thrilled that in the chronically oversharing age of social media, and despite advances in surgery and product technology, Hollywood has retained some smoke and mirror effects. With nothing more than a square of sticky paper.

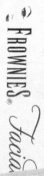

FROWNIES® *Facial*

for wrinkles on the Forehea

Smooth wrinkles while you sleep
· soften facial expressions
· look younger by relaxing expression li

144 patches

8–16 week supply

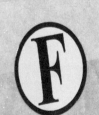

When I was about seven, my grandmother and I took the bus into town and walked down to Pino's Salon for a set. Having thus far been raised by a single dad who took my brothers and me to Tommy's barbershop every couple of months and asked for three identical haircuts, I'd never before been to a ladies' salon. Lined up in little chairs, in a room no bigger than the lounge in a council house, were half a dozen older ladies, their hair wrapped around convex curlers, secured tightly with white rubber bands, and hidden underneath domed dryers like pixies in acorn hats. As they flicked through dog-eared copies of *Woman's Own*, they talked of the Home Secretary William Whitelaw, I remember, and of Marti Caine's weight, and of someone's husband suspected to be living a secret double life. All this was shouted over the whirr of dryers, while Pino, an ostensibly Italian man with an implausible accent (even to a child) and dressed at least thirty years too young, minced around with a tail comb, making them all laugh.

I can remember almost every detail of Pino's Salon, but what I couldn't quite describe until I discovered Boots Essentials Pink Curl Crème some twenty-eight years later, was the smell – strongly perfumed but so comforting and feminine that it narrowly swerves 'cloying' (though my very happy memory may be positively skewing my reaction). Nonetheless, Curl Crème is a bloody marvellous little bargain and should be owned by anyone with naturally curly hair. It's a thick, pearlescent gunk one rakes sparingly through wet curls (use too much and it goes crunchy) with fingertips or a wide-tooth comb, before drying either naturally or in a diffuser attachment. It stops frizz, adds great definition, and comes in a pleasingly no-frills plastic tub that lasts for ages. It's silicone-free but does contain alcohol, so can be pretty drying on the hair if used too often, and should be counterbalanced with plenty of deep-conditioning treatments. It's enjoyed something of a revival thanks to the Curlygirl Movement (do Google – it's marvellously useful), but as someone with pin-straight hair I own it purely for the scent. One whiff and I'm back at Pino's, sitting on a pile of telephone books, praying never to return to my dad's barbershop and thinking how much nicer it is to be a girl.

essentials

curl
crème

natural
control and defines

It's a cause of some sadness to me that I've never been a blonde. I just feel too connected to my brunette status, too entrenched in my self-identity, to ever take the plunge. But when I do allow myself to fantasise, I am always the kind of cool, Hitchcock heroine blonde that requires Touch of Silver brightening shampoo. This, a beauty classic, uses sheer purple tones to counteract brassiness and add brightness and shine to grey, silver or bleached blonde hair (despite the alarming colour of the gel, it does not turn hair a fetching shade of Mrs Slocombe lilac, perhaps more's the pity). It's cheap, available in every town and is, in my experience, the brightening shampoo most often recommended by hairdressers.

It is not as unique as it once was – there are now very good versions across all price points (Aveda Blue Malva and the excellent sulphate-free Joico Violet shampoos, for example) – but Touch of Silver deserves special recognition because in 1977 it was the first haircare brand designed purely to enhance grey and white hair, not to cover or disguise it (its significant benefits to bleached blonde hair were an accidental by-product). When women had always been told to stave off the ageing process no matter what, Touch of Silver encouraged them not only to embrace it, but to find the unique beauty in growing older. It didn't ignore our nanas when they were apparently invisible to the rest of the industry. It's hard to imagine now, when even very young women are dyeing their hair silver and white, how subversive a message that was, but in its own small, unpretentious way, Touch of Silver shifted beauty an inch in the right direction.

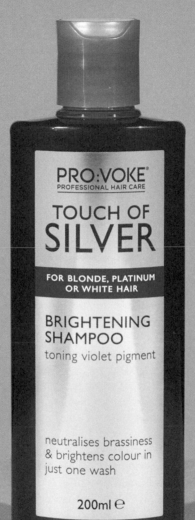

It's ironic that 4711 should appear in the Nostalgics section when, at time of writing, colognes are again proving so popular and cool. I'm thrilled to see it, but then cologne never left my pulse points. These are very light, citrusy (usually from lemon and bergamot) and crisp fragrances which, despite smelling to me like a fresh ironing pile in a fancy French hotel, were born in Cologne, Germany. It's widely believed that 4711, launched in 1792 (and worn by Napoleon), was the first of them – which makes it all the more wonderful and amazing that you still buy it in Boots for under a tenner. Like most colognes, 4711 (initially named Aqua Mirabilis, meaning Wonder Water) is a fresh, fleeting, ostensibly unisex but primarily male fragrance that acts as the perfect transitional scent for late summer, or for year-round use as a light first layer over which to spray a stronger, longer lasting perfume. It's also, in my experience, the perfect response to those who claim to hate perfume, as it's so polite, jolly and unobtrusive and (more elegantly) mimics the smell of shower-drenched hair and skin. But 4711 is more than just the definitive example of its genre, it's a statement of intent.

At the beginning of the film *Breakfast at Tiffany's*, heroine Audrey Hepburn as Holly Golightly gets ready to visit a rich gangster in prison, while George Peppard's Paul Varjak looks on in awe. We see her brush her teeth, fix her hair in a chignon, put on an enormous black hat. She is breathtakingly stylish. Before they leave, she opens her tiny mailbox at the front door of her Manhattan apartment, reaches into it and pulls out an anonymous perfume atomiser and spritzes her neck, then applies a perfect shade of coral lipstick. It's a gorgeous, elegant scene in a wonderful film, but one that's always frustrated me enormously, because in the original novella by Truman Capote we read that Holly wears 4711. To me, the fact that this flighty, rather messed-up and fragile girl wears such a bright, unpretentious, confident and inexpensive men's cologne is an insightful to the point of crucial observation, and adds another dimension to a character I've always found ever so slightly annoying (I realise this is considered by many to be sacrilege).

Perfume reveals so much about a person's self-image, and *Breakfast at Tiffany's* filmmakers – so otherwise meticulous in their depiction of personal style – missed a trick and sold her short. Literary Holly, in her 4711 cologne, is so much more complex than Hollywood Holly, who wears some expensive-looking, feminine scent that could be worn by any New York café society geisha. And these, I'm afraid, are the things that keep me awake in my bed.

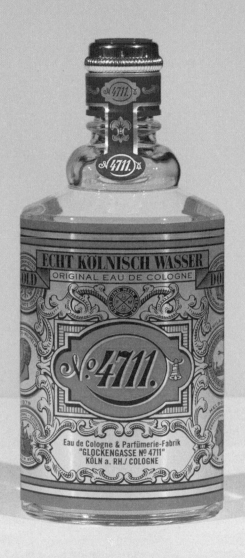

I am generally suspicious of multitasking products. They seem like a lovely idea but dual lip and cheek colours are often gorgeous and dewy on the face, chalky and dull on the mouth. Shampoo and conditioner combis typically leave hair lank and a bit sad-looking, 2-in-1 moisturisers and primers fail to deliver on either brief and so on. Besides, I love beauty products and unless I one day find myself on a camping trip (my marrying Donald Trump is only marginally less likely), my preference is generally for more, not fewer, potions.

But Dr Bronner's pure-Castile soap is my one very cheerful concession to multitasking. It's a high-quality, natural, liquid wash – unchanged since 1908 – invented for the purposes of washing: hands, hair, clothes (especially the handwashing of jumpers, where it's excellent), babies, worktops, toys and dishes. Its no-nasties formula even allows it to act as a safe toothpaste substitute in an emergency (the peppermint and coconut 'flavours' are best for this). It's made by a family-run company founded by Dr Emanuel Bronner, a German-Jewish, third-generation master soapmaker under the guild system of the time. The brand is eco-friendly, cruelty-free and heavily invested in fairtrade schemes, organic farming, charities and ethical workplace practices. It's therefore especially satisfying that without any major advertising, and with a mostly independent health food and gift shop distribution, Dr Bronner's beautifully simple colour-coded bottles of liquid soap now sell at a rate of about 11 million per year.

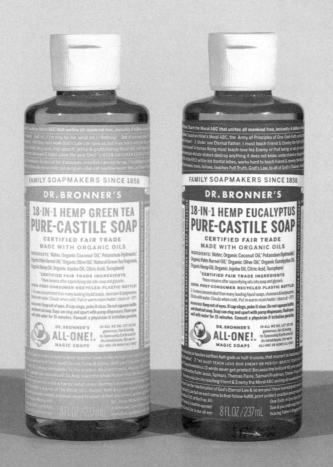

At time of writing, I have worked in the beauty industry for almost twenty-five years, tested countless products for every conceivable skin type or problem, researched many thousands of brands, and I still don't really understand what the bloody hell Erno Laszlo skincare is all about. And I must confess that this is exactly why I sort of love it. This large and somewhat baffling skincare range was devised by Hungarian dermatologist Laszlo in the 1920s to use on his client base of Hungarian princesses and movie stars. He soon moved on to Hollywood, where he focused on improving the complexions of the studio system's biggest actresses such as Ava Gardner, Katharine Hepburn and Grace Kelly.

He opened up a private practice too, nicknamed 'The House of Silence' by client Wallis Simpson, referring to all the secrets within, and launched fifteen products at Saks Fifth Avenue. Uniquely in an industry then fixated on wrinkle creams, Laszlo was way ahead of his time in putting greater focus on cleansing ('I taught the high-society ladies in America to wash their face,' he once boasted), particularly with solid bars of black mud face soap, as featured and namechecked in Woody Allen's Oscar-winning *Annie Hall*.

There are few brands in history to enjoy such widespread and devoted celebrity endorsement as Erno Laszlo. Katharine Hepburn and Jackie Kennedy were fans, and Garbo continued to see Laszlo long after she withdrew from public life. Audrey Hepburn once attributed 50 per cent of her beauty to her mother, '50 per cent to Erno Laszlo'. Chillingly, a jar of Erno Laszlo Active Phelityl Cream can even be seen next to Marilyn Monroe's bed in police photography taken shortly after her death (the pair were good friends, and Laszlo had created Phormula especially for her).

Erno Laszlo products – Phelityl, Phormula and cleansing bars included – are still available worldwide. They are expensive (a hundred-odd quid for a night cream), have finally ditched their brilliant but wilfully retro marbled packaging, and are too numerous and confusing to buy without full consultation. They also mostly contain mineral oil and/or alcohol, possibly because the brand daren't reformulate or modernise products so deeply loved by its loyal, borderline evangelical, clientele. But in terms of old Hollywood glamour, legend and mystique, I don't think any product line could ever hope to equal Laszlo's. They are iconic products loved and endorsed by some of the most iconic women of all time.

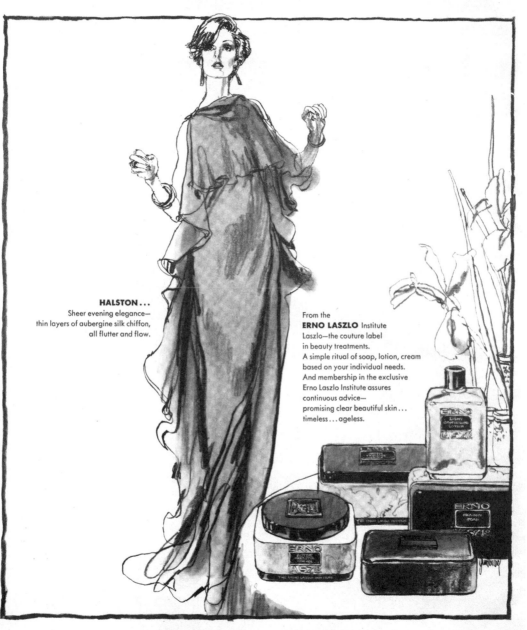

HALSTON...
Sheer evening elegance—
thin layers of aubergine silk chiffon,
all flutter and flow.

From the
ERNO LASZLO Institute
Laszlo—the couture label
in beauty treatments.
A simple ritual of soap, lotion, cream
based on your individual needs.
And membership in the exclusive
Erno Laszlo Institute assures
continuous advice—
promising clear beautiful skin...
timeless...ageless.

Mabel·Danahy
BUFFALO, NEW YORK

CELEBRATING FIFTY YEARS OF FASHION

I'm asked often if I'd one day like my own product range and while I wouldn't be so presumptuous as to anticipate any future opportunity, my mind does wander to what I would do with it. But I rarely get beyond what jewellery designer and cubist heiress Paloma Picasso did in the eighties: one signature perfume, one beautifully packaged red lipstick in a heavy gold tube, one matching nail polish. I confess I have a weakness for brands that make only a small number of things, and I admire the confidence and chutzpah here in offering just one shade – a blueish red that Paloma Picasso apparently wore to 'keep people away'. Which, of course, is another reason I loved the Paloma Picasso brand. It was red. I have written acres of copy on red lipstick at this point and so I'm sure regular readers more than get the gist. But in the conception of Mon Rouge, Picasso summed up what makes red lipstick so unique.

Much is made of make-up's dishonesty, its pretence that skin is flawless, lashes are long, cheekbones sharp. Its talent for disguise, illusion and conformity is held up as the reason it's so corrupting and unfeminist. But red lipstick is quite the opposite. No one's lips are naturally crimson – it has no pretensions and makes no attempt at realism. Far from selling out to attract the opposite sex, it actively discourages advances from those not man enough to take on the inevitable colour transfer and smudging – not to mention whichever strong personality opted to wear it. Red lipstick, while utterly sexy, chic, stylish and glamorous, exists primarily for the woman wearing it, not for the people beholding it, making it the most feminist make-up item of all. It's uncompromising, powerful and demands to be noticed.

Sadly, I never owned Mon Rouge, and have subsequently tried intermittently, and failed, to get one in good second-hand condition (only the perfume is still in production). But it's probably fitting that I only got to admire it on the pages of my mum's glossy magazines. Its price tag – a whopping £15 when Clinique was around £6 – and intimidating maturity kept me away. Which was Paloma's intention, I'm sure.

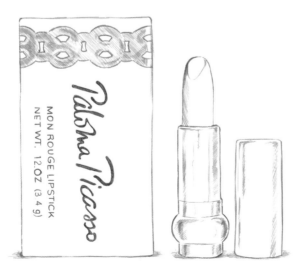

MON ROUGE LIPSTICK
NET WT. 12.OZ (3.4 g)

Paloma Picasso

The Christmas manicure kit is for those whose personality has proved too indistinct, too unremarkable, for a more thoughtful or apposite present. It's a mock-croc, gold-tone, clip-shut, hard-case wallet containing jagged nail clippers, scissors that could barely cut butter, and a metal file so brutal that your nails may never fully recover from the courtesy-demo. It is the beauty equivalent of petrol station flowers, sold in pound shops, department store gift sections, chemists with not much else on offer. In recent years, the Christmas manicure kit has seen a decline in popularity, losing out to the Victoriana shaving stand, complete with faux ivory barbershop brush and ye olde mahogany-handled razor with Mach 3 head. But it lacks the nana-like charm of the original and costs about eight times as much.

My grandmother wore Yardley English Lavender every single day and probably for this reason alone it remains the only lavender smell I love (I can't bear its prominence in almost everything else – those lavender-filled sleeping masks are quite literally the stuff of nightmares). Born before the Great War (Yardley itself has been around since 1770) and made from neroli, geranium, patchouli, vanilla and lavender grown in Kent, Yardley's scent is soft, warm, soothing almost to the point of soporific, and, I think, rather elegant. It's relatively affordable and sold alongside toiletries in old-fashioned chemists next to throat lozenges and cough syrup, or in Mother's Day gift packs with matching hand cream and soap.

It's the kind of perfume normal British women of my nan's generation wore – the women who worked in offices and munitions factories, who simultaneously cared for their families with ration coupons and very little money, and to whom French scents from Chanel or Dior were as alien and untouchable as mangoes for tea. Its modest lack of pretension, pomp or ceremony is one of the things I love most about English Lavender and about Yardley generally. To me it is a fireside cuddle, my nose pressed into my nan's apron as she shelled peas, or a game of gin rummy, her scent wafting over the little card table. It's the kind of unmistakably British perfume that might sweep past in a foreign land and cause an immediate pang of homesickness. It's delicious, no-nonsense, polite and refined.

Sadly, Yardley English Lavender was reformulated and relaunched in March 2015, and its new incarnation, while perfectly pleasant, is less evocative of the sturdy, stoic women who once wore it. I respect Yardley's need to modernise, of course. A brand of such standing and commitment deserves to represent more than just nostalgia. I am happy that Yardley exists, and fearful it won't always. The fact that it continues to manufacture exclusively in Britain, even though scarcely anyone else does and it's costing the company a great deal to do so, is just one of many reasons to support it in its programme of modernisation. Yardley received a cash injection from the Middle East a few years ago (I'm delighted someone saved it), but in every other respect this iconic house remains as British as Victoria sponge. Do revisit its wares.

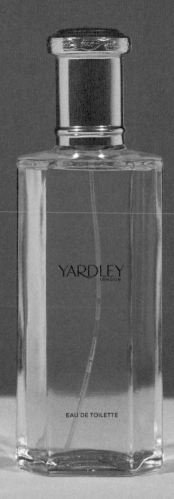

In 1932, in the midst of America's Great Depression, nail polish came in only pale or transparent shades. Identifying an opportunity, brothers Charles and Joseph Revson enlisted the help of chemist Charles Lachman to create Cherries in the Snow, the first ever opaque coloured nail enamel in bold pinky red, and set about selling it door to door. A few years later, Charles Revson spotted a woman in a restaurant wearing mismatched lipstick and nail polish, and so he decided to make a lip shade to match perfectly each of his now large array of nail colours. Cherries in the Snow lipstick was born.

Revson's 'Matching Lips & Tips' concept took off to such a degree that it has only really fallen out of fashion in the last decade or two. I personally love a mismatch – red lips with orange or hot pink nails, and vice versa – but there is something brilliantly Alexis Carrington Colby about a matching red mouth and talons, and so I can't resist the occasional nod to Revson's vision. His Revlon company still has arguably the most classic, recognisable reds in the entire beauty industry.

Revlon Red, born soon after Cherries in the Snow, is the brand's most iconic, and is about as true a Marilyn Monroe red as one can find anywhere. Fire & Ice, launched in 1952, is the equally cool-toned, slightly corally counterpoint to Cherries in the Snow and my personal favourite – not least because it was the shade worn by my dear friend Carey Lander, who elevated the wearing of bold lipstick to something of an art form. While a collector of Chanel, Tom Ford, Rimmel London, Lancôme and many more, she favoured Revlon's simple, affordable black and gold tubes and vintage-style creamy formulation overall. Fire & Ice was the lipstick she wore throughout chemotherapy, the lipstick she so often wore on stage to play keyboards and sing, the shade she painted on when she felt dreadful, poorly, happy, mischievous, despairing and as celebratory as someone so laconic and pithy could ever be.

I so closely associate her with the colour that when Carey died in 2015, I decided I'd like guests at her funeral to each take home a tube of Fire & Ice. Having cleared out three branches of Boots and with still nowhere near enough to give those bereft of someone so hugely popular, I contacted Revlon to place a very large rush order of Fire & Ice and Revlon Red. They delivered hundreds of lipsticks in a matter of days. While I'm under absolutely no illusions about my position of professional privilege, and my consequent access to brands (I am beyond grateful for both), I am also privy to how cut-throat the beauty industry can be. Editors made redundant from their once influential jobs suddenly find themselves knocked off guest lists after years of supporting a brand. Once close relationships follow the same trajectory as a failing magazine's circulation.

Few acts of kindness occur purely for their own sake. And so I was touched deeply by Revlon's elegant insistence that this was for Carey, not for publicity. They didn't want me to write about it, they have never once reminded me of it, hinted at a reciprocal favour, or frankly even shown much enthusiasm for their inclusion in this book. They just wanted to mark the passing of an utterly memorable woman with one of their most iconic shades of red. They, and Carey, were class acts. Sadly, I'm not, and so I've chosen to ignore their wishes.

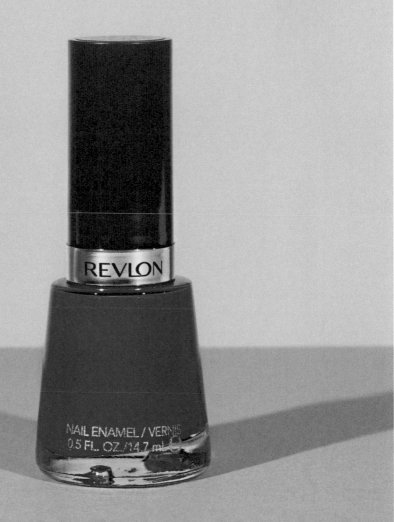

A pressed cube of perfumed Epsom salts, wrapped in foil paper and adorned with a paper band featuring an illustration of the Swiss Alps, Kew Garden hydrangeas, or some quiet scene on the lawn at York Minster, boxed in batches of nine and sold in the sort of gift shops where one might also find Dundee marmalade, scone recipe tea towels and vinyl bookmarks in a fetching shade of maroon. The idea was that the bath cube was unsheathed from its souvenir packaging, then plopped into a running bath to dissolve, scent and soften the water, turning mundane bath times into something exciting and posh.

Except that the peculiar thing about bath cubes is that no one seemed ever to buy them, even from the National Trust gift shops they inhabited. They just sort of appeared in people's homes, via the endlessly recycled spare present drawers of Britain's nans, like some black market operated by the silver-haired mafia. Whenever someone unexpected dropped by over Christmas, my own beloved grandmother, Nance, would nip upstairs and grab some dusty bath cubes from the under-bed archive, which I imagined were then stored in the recipient's own smellies drawer to be similarly recycled next year. And so on, until the Christmas my grandmother would ultimately get them back, boxes bruised but still emitting potent lily of the valley. Then I might get to have one fizzing half-heartedly around my Sunday night bath, turning to gritty sludge on my leg, filling the tiny bathroom with the smell of stewed petals. There was nothing more decadent, and no greater treat, and if you look back at bath cubes with similar affection, do look on eBay. Their shelf life is almost infinite, their vintage packaging even more beautiful than I remembered, their cost so low that you'll be hard pushed to stop. The only sadness is imagining which nana is no longer in need of her present drawer.

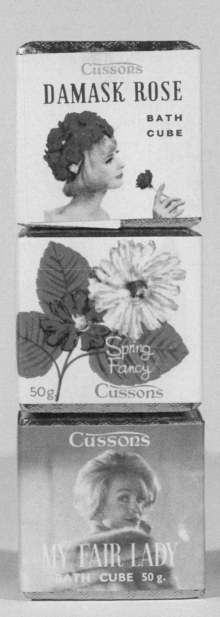

A few years ago, I became an Avon lady for the day, and discovered that the old, if charming, stereotype of some suburban Stepford Wife in a pillbox hat, tottering door-to-door to flog lipsticks like double glazing, is dead and buried. Things have moved on since I was a little girl obsessed with make-up and the local Avon ladies in my South Wales valleys community. Avon ladies (and often men) now are students, single parents, rural farmers, retired career women, entrepreneurs, or simply those looking to combine a fun social life with earning some extra cash.

Founder David H. McConnell pioneered the idea of a women-only door-to-door sales model in 1886, offering complete flexibility of working hours and financial independence before American women even had the vote. Today, Avon has 6.5 million reps worldwide, all managing themselves. One in three women in the UK is an Avon customer and 6 million British women see an Avon brochure every three weeks. To fill the pages, Avon (whose motto is 'The Company for Women') develops a staggering 1,000 new products per year – an unprecedented output from a beauty brand – from its own research and development laboratories in the US. They are perfectly serviceable (and appear to inspire almost zealous devotion from customers, who seem reluctant to even consider using anything else) and often cheaper than many supermarket own-brand labels.

Being an Avon lady is hardly going to make someone the next Anita Roddick. But that doesn't make Avon an irrelevance, nor the women involved mere hobbyists. This small business opportunity gives very many women the first money they've ever earned independently – earnings they can spend as they please, or contribute financially to their marriages and family for the first time.

And besides, to measure the value of Avon reps by the money they make is to miss the point entirely. All the Avon ladies I've spoken to know a great number of their neighbours by name, and speak of the older customers they call on for a cuppa purely to make sure they receive at least one visitor that week. Many reps regularly hand out free samples to 'mature ladies' because they know their pensions are too meagre for any frivolous purchases beyond the odd bottle of talcum powder. One rep I met in Brighton returns to one customer more regularly than is commercially worthwhile because she fears for her client's safety within a physically abusive marriage (domestic violence was Avon's main charitable cause before people really talked about it). Other women may have lost confidence in their personal appearance after children or menopause. Some customers have such poor mobility that they rely on Avon to prevent them from becoming isolated from the outside world.

It's easy to dismiss Avon, and, more widely, beauty products, as an irrelevance, but no other industry can boast such an all-embracing army of empowered women working flexible hours, often from their own homes and serving their local communities, whether or not that effort results in a couple more pounds in the kitty. And having spent time within this unique and supportive workforce, there is absolutely no doubt in my mind that many Avon reps are doing so much more than selling make-up – they're providing an unlikely, but crucial, community service. I hope Avon celebrates its next century with pride.

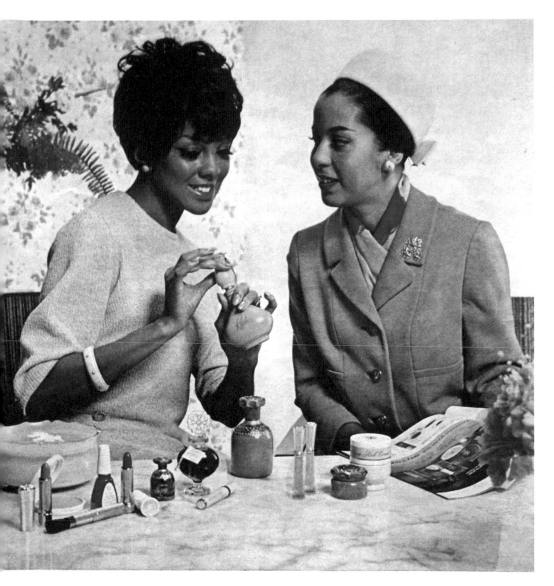

The Art of being a Woman:
An interest You and your Avon Representative share

Beauty is important to your neighborly Avon Representative. How to put on makeup, what's new in color, fashion, complexion care—these are her interests, too. Every day your Avon Representative perfects the art of being a woman, at home. Then, when she calls on you—she shares her time and knowledge with you. She always brings beauty ideas, cosmetics and fragrances to please you. So take a little time for yourself. Have an Avon beauty chat.

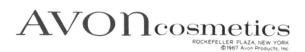

AVON cosmetics

ROCKEFELLER PLAZA, NEW YORK
©1967 Avon Products, Inc.

When I read wistful food books describing the citrus fruits of Tuscan or Provence markets, I always think the British equivalent is stumbling across an independent chemist with a faded window display, chiming door, locked cabinet of Kent combs and Mason Pearson hairbrushes, and a table of tissue-wrapped Bronnley lemons and limes, scenting the air with their soft, soapy zest. You don't find it anything like enough these days, which is why, when my friend India and I experienced exactly this scene while on holiday in Southwold three summers ago, we squealed with happiness and each bought several boxes.

The soaps themselves are of a lovely quality, as one might expect from the Queen's soap maker – triple milled and with added moisturising shea butter, convincingly coloured and fashioned into fruits – but the appeal of Bronnley is for me mostly sentimental. As a little girl, I loved receiving their special Easter soap in its pretty egg-shaped tin, and simply cannot remember a time when the fruit soaps didn't exist (Bronnley has been making them since 1892, when James Bronnley was inspired by the increasing number of exotic fruits becoming available to British people). They are the never-to-be-used display soaps of a British guest bathroom, the jewel in the crown of my nan's emergency present drawer, an eccentric and jolly British icon that I hope will never be retired.

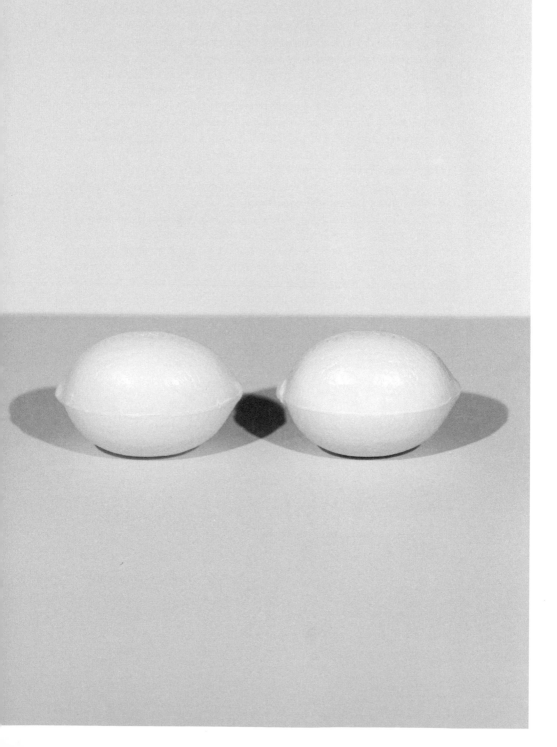

For me, Penhaligon's Bluebell is more than a beauty icon, it's ostensibly a perfume for the kind of woman I'll never be. Its image is soft, quaint, innocent, restrained and effortlessly cool. It's for the kind of woman who finds a priceless Ossie Clark dress in a Sue Ryder shop, who can wear a skinny vest and no bra without chafing, who looks great in nothing but clear mascara and a brisk pinch of the cheeks, and who can achieve casual, surfer-girl waves without forty-five minutes wrestling with tongs. Its very pretty, grosgrain ribbon-tied apothecary bottle and powder-blue jus imply old age, but Bluebell is surprisingly young. It was launched in 1978 and accessorised rather perfectly the cheesecloth smocks and floral pie-crust-collared maxi dresses of the day. It quickly developed a loyal following (it's expensive at a little shy of a hundred quid a bottle and so will always be a cult rather than a celebrity) and sold consistently, but became especially relevant again thanks to the bohemian fashion resurgence in the early 2000s – yet another good reason for me not to wear it (be grateful that you've never had to see me in fringed suede).

And yet oddly, the scent within doesn't quite fit its exterior image. It does – at least, to my nose – smell of wild bluebells. But they're more earthy and wet than they are floral and sweet, even with the touch of English rose and hyacinth to even things out. There's a soft spiciness here too, thanks to cinnamon and clove, that stops the whole thing feeling too Laura Ashley and twee. But there's also a bitterness overall, which one either loves or hates. Kate Moss, who apparently wore it on her wedding day, loves it. As did Princess Diana. But most tellingly, perhaps, is the fact that Margaret Thatcher adored Bluebell. Like Thatcher, I find this scent is pretending to be demure and feminine, when in fact it's a tad harsh and lingers far longer than you'd like.

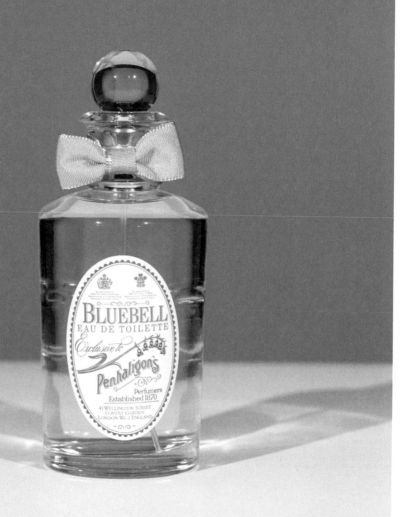

I have a great love for compacts generally. They are chic, polite, the kind of accessory that would now be as outmoded as hat, gloves and cigarette case if it weren't for the fact that, as humans, we will never tire of gazing at ourselves in the mirror. Mrs Estée Lauder loved them too and in 1963 she began producing collectable powder or perfume compacts, often designing them herself, to gift to dinner party guests and sell in small quantities to customers. Instead of the classic round compact design carried by every woman, these were novelty items, inspired by everything from a perfectly formed seashell found on the beach at Lauder's Florida home, to Victorian pillboxes brought back from her trips to Europe. Like antiques and artworks, the compacts caught the eye of collectors, and soon Estée Lauder began releasing new compacts each year, date stamping each and limiting designs to a single release, available while stocks lasted. It's a rather pleasing beauty industry tradition that survives to this day, long after Mrs Lauder's passing.

But the reason I so love Estée Lauder's collectable compacts is that the thousands of collectors worldwide are simply my people. Some people collect stamps, or wine, or football cards. These people stalk eBay, antique fairs and junk shops for weird and rare powder compacts then display them in glass cabinets purely for their own pleasure. These obsessive make-up collectors would understand why I have every special edition Stila eyeshadow palette since 1997, why I have approximately 370 rosy-beige lipsticks with barely a whisper of a difference between each, why I have at least four lip balms in each handbag, and why I'd sooner give away valuables than I would a shade from the YSL La Laque Couture nail polish back catalogue. They'd understand why I cried when my Ultima II: The Nakeds blusher cracked upon falling from the shelf, why I can never throw out a perfume bottle.

And so while I am not personally turned on by whimsical compacts, moulded and enamelled to look like ladybirds, teddy bears, zodiac signs, fairground carousels and the Leaning Tower of Pisa, I am comforted by the existence of those who are, and by Estée Lauder's insistence on continuing to release new designs each year, and on ensuring that the correct refills of Lucidity powder or solid perfume remain available. They are elegant, somewhat eccentric items with a sense of history and permanence in a wasteful and disposable culture. I like nerds, I love beauty nerds even more, and I admire Estée Lauder for looking after them.

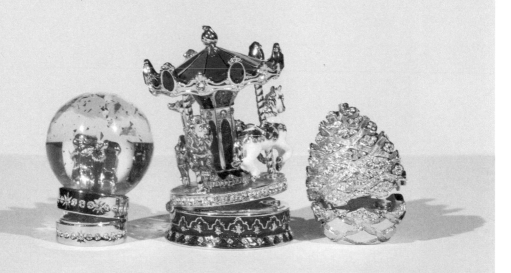

I wish I was the kind of woman who used cuticle cream. Who sits, brushing her hair, in an oyster silk kimono at her ornate dressing table, shooing away the dashing husband kissing her neck so she can tend to her nails in peace. This is always how I imagine the owner of Crème Abricot, Dior's legendary cuticle treatment packaged in a relatively unchanged, vintage monogrammed pot which – perhaps surprisingly in a modern world – still sells by the hundredweight. I have no use for Crème Abricot, neither the time nor the inclination for it, and yet I covet a life that affords the maintenance of cuticles and the slow caressing of necks. And so I keep a pot in the drawer, in case of seismic shift.

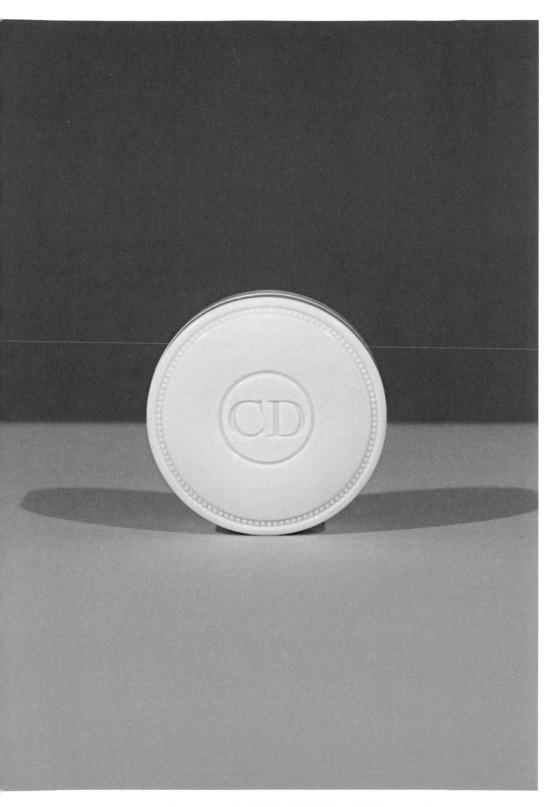

Your typical 1970s travel brochure: a cover featuring a toned and carefree family, frolicking in the surf, and page after page of gleaming, new-build hotels towering behind suspiciously blue and empty-deckchair-surrounded pools. Your typical 1970s holiday? Not, as the saying goes, like the brochure. Seven a.m. deckchair raids. Trying to make an Orangina last an hour and a paperback last the week. Gingerly guiding your flip-flops through unidentified liquids on the floor of the pungent public beachside bogs. Waiting three days for an English paper. And as far as the sweat-stinging eye could see, bodies slowly sizzling in a Coppertone marinade.

Coppertone's roots actually lie in the US military. Benjamin Green, a Florida pharmacist and Second World War airman, used a concoction called Red Veterinary Petroleum (mmm, sounds lovely) to protect himself and his colleagues from the sun. Before the war was even over, Green had blended the 'red vet pet' with cocoa butter and coconut and created a rudimentary form of the lotion with which generations of holidaymakers would leave sun loungers impregnated for decades to come.

The brand really took off thanks to a 1959 advertising campaign which introduced the Coppertone Girl, a blonde toddler illustrated in the act of having her bikini bottoms removed by a pesky cocker spaniel and revealing an untanned bum. The character has endured in various iterations – 3-year-old Jodie Foster's acting debut came in a 1965 Coppertone ad, and today the Coppertone Girl has her modesty preserved by a dress.

The science of suncream has, thankfully, advanced considerably since the war, with waterproofing and the gradual refinement of UVA and UVB protection proving particularly welcome. These changes have in part been heralded by the descendants of Benjamin Green's original sunscreen formula, but for me Coppertone really is all about the age of the package holiday, when the browner you looked, the healthier it was assumed you were, and protection from the sun was a secondary concern. It speaks of a time when summer meant fly and fry.

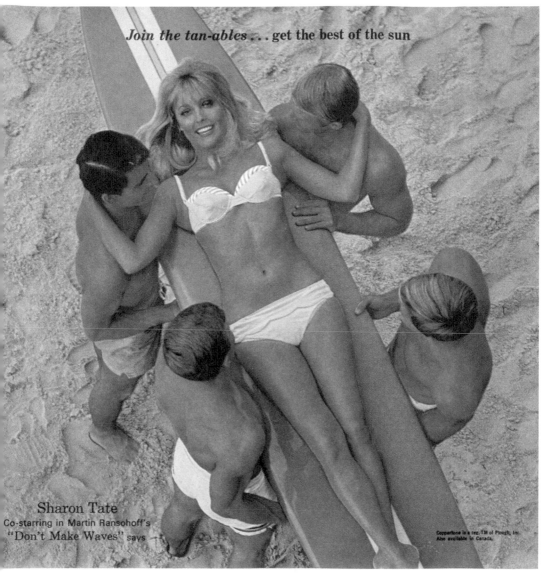

I adore Pears, but could just as easily have chosen Imperial Leather, Camay (recently, and quite unexpectedly, bought by Unilever and soon to return to the shelves), Wright's moisture-stripping Coal Tar or eighties macho classic, Shield. Retro soaps are the most evocative products of all to me. They're the blanket smell of my childhood: my stepfather coming in to wash his hands with a stripy, oil-smeared tablet of Shield after fixing the constantly malfunctioning car; my mother dropping a bar of Pears into a bowl of warm water to sponge-wash the baby's bum; the smell of the flannels my grandmother pre-soaped with Imperial Leather for when I got up for school; my grandad rubbing dry Wright's across his hair to set it.

Nowadays I receive beautiful, moisturising liquid handwashes from Molton Brown or L'Occitane, or buy from a wall of generic anti-bac pumps in the supermarket, and feel momentarily saddened that solid household soap has become such a superannuated novelty. Even at Number 10 Downing Street, where one might fairly expect an old-school ablution, I found a grubby bottle of Carex in place of the coat of arms-branded, tissue-wrapped soap tablet I'd hoped to steal. But for generations of people – myself included – good, old-fashioned soaps were, and notionally remain, lovely, fatty, sweet, lanolin-rich bars of daily British life.

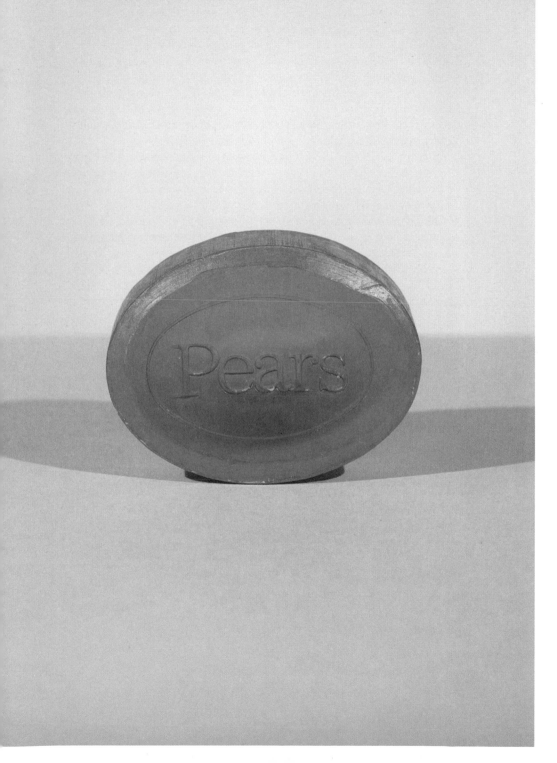

My 6-year-old self felt the Stratton to be the pinnacle of womanhood. It was a sturdy, non-precious metal compact, sold in several designs at independent pharmacies and dusty old department stores, into which one could click any standard face powder refill, like Rimmel Stay Matte or Max Factor Creme Puff. Each Stratton ('of Mayfair', don't you know) came in a little velvet handbag pouch and gift box, making it a popular working- to lower-middle-class choice for landmark birthday, anniversary and retirement gifts. Strattons aren't posh in the luxury, moneyed sense. An aristocrat or design snob would probably sneer at them. Personally, I adore them (I own four, plus one of their enamelled lipstick cases) and everything they represent.

A Stratton compact is the kind of high-quality, practical, no-nonsense item owned by British ladies who are girl scout leaders, secretaries and members of the WI (my grandmother was all three), who could change a fan belt or rewire a tea urn whenever required. It belonged in a deceptively capacious handbag alongside a spare fuse, emergency sewing kit and two dozen safety pins. During stuffier times, it afforded its owner a degree of respectability; one could powder one's nose from a Stratton without appearing vain or gauche, then click it shut in the firm, businesslike manner of an accountant shutting his briefcase. Stratton of Mayfair is a noble, charming British business, and I am extremely comforted by its continued existence at John Lewis, House of Fraser and in independent chemists nationwide. Do support them.

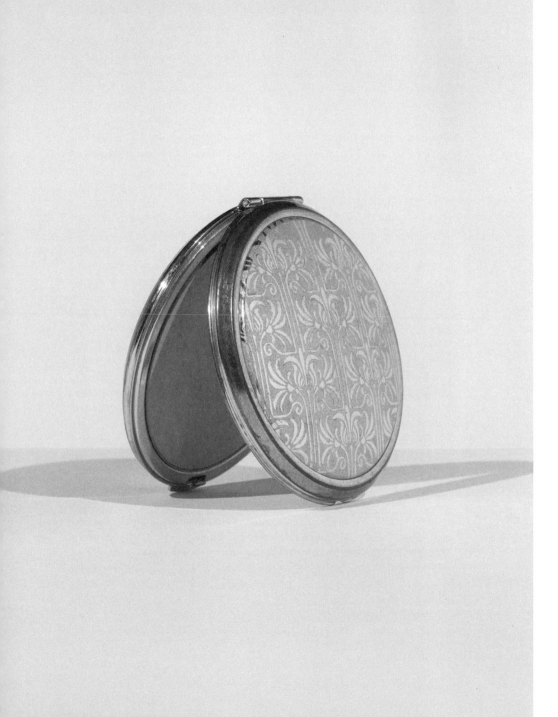

It's true to say that the process of creating a celebrity perfume usually goes something like this: celebrity is approached by fragrance companies, who pitch to agents and managers for the exclusive licence to create the star's own perfume. A company is chosen and briefed by celebrity's agent (small chance of celebrity themselves attending briefing meetings). Company makes around five perfumes in response to brief and presents to agent. Celebrity reliably picks one that smells like air freshener and cupcake frosting. Company designs three bottles. Celebrity picks one. Celebrity turns up at promotional photo shoot and press conference citing childhood garden/favourite holiday destination/kindly grandmother/love of life as inspiration. Public buys. Celebrity and agent contemplate sequel.

Yes, I am cynical. But not even 1 per cent as cynical as celebrity perfumery as an exercise. One of the few exceptions is Elizabeth Taylor, who invented the modern concept of 'celebrity perfume' and demonstrated a lasting passion for, and interest in, her product far more profound than most of the dimmer (interpret as you wish) stars who followed in her wake. Taylor shrewdly partnered with Elizabeth Arden to create her collection of eleven perfumes, kicking off with Passion in 1987, and supervised each of them, even in failing health (her last perfume, Violet Eyes, was released only a year before her death). Her genuine attachment to the range was reflected in the fact she always wore her own creation – White Diamonds.

White Diamonds is all about flower power: a florgasm of lily, neroli and bergamot underpinned by violet, jasmine, rose, ylang ylang, narcissus and tuberose, the whole bouquet arranged in a sturdy pot of amber, sandalwood and oak moss. Like the rest of Taylor's olfactory output, White Diamonds is not to everyone's taste. Richard Burton's observation that Taylor was 'too bloody much' could just as accurately have been levelled at her portfolio of big, ball-breaking statement scents. They pulled no punches and made few concessions to modernity, even when the trend for insipid unisex fragrances dominated the market in the nineties.

The perfume's clean, candy right hook certainly landed: White Diamonds was an instant success, doing $35 million worth of business in its first season. Not that this success at the tills was unrepresentative – the lion's share of Taylor's $600 million fortune came not from her film work, but her perfumes.

Unsurprisingly, when Taylor passed away in 2011, Elizabeth Arden was quick to announce the range would not die with her. Confident, uncompromising and unambiguous, the qualities Taylor's perfumes share with their creator allow them to act, alongside her extraordinary body of work, as a vibrant testament to true Hollywood star quality.

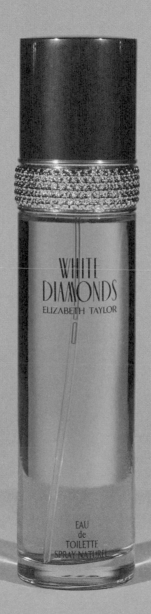

In unpredictable times, there's something doughty and dependable about the simple soap bar. It's comforting, economical and, it turns out, less drying than it used to be. Nowadays, quality soaps are frequently triple-milled, which makes for a more durable, sudsy bar that retains its integrity down to the last sliver, instead of retiring gloopily into the depths of the soap dish.

Of course the soap bar still comes in myriad forms and runs the full gamut from those ephemeral, paper-wrapped Milky Bar offcuts which are the sole preserve of hotel bathrooms, to the pretty, floral-paper-wrapped offerings you'll find in high-end department stores.

And at that desirable end of the soap spectrum, you'll find Marseille soap. Marseille soap, which has been produced in the region since the fourteenth century, is traditionally made by mixing Mediterranean sea water with olive oil, soda ash and lye.

L'Occitane's Bonne Mère is a Marseille soap presented in delightfully modest square blocks of multi-flavoured goodness. The blocks are made with at least 72 per cent olive oil (and eco-friendly palm oil) and they're as handy for scenting a drawer and washing the clothes within it as they are for cleaning the wearer. And of course they're lovely and tactile – running fingertips over the debossed lettering on the front of a fresh block is a sensation no basin-side pump bottle can dream of offering.

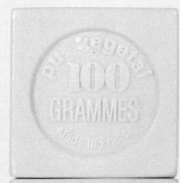
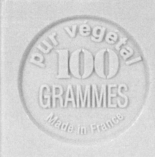
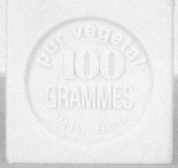

It is endlessly saddening that I was born too late to go shopping at Big Biba, the seven-storey Kensington High Street department store opened by Barbara Hulanicki in 1973. The elaborate, Willy Wonka-esque store sold everything from tinned sardines and dog food to mini dresses and ice buckets, but Biba beauty, which strongly referenced 1920s Hollywood glamour, combining it with sixties mod doe-eyes and seventies disco glitter, was arguably the most influential on how we shop today. Biba sold glamorous, luxury make-up to the masses: nail polishes and lip glosses were as cheap as they were covetable, and stacked on a self-selection counter rather than produced by a department store clerk from locked, inaccessible drawers (think the Benefit and Smashbox counters of today, with prices closer to Rimmel and Bourjois). Biba was the first shopping environment to allow women to try on 'testers' of beauty products without committing themselves to a purchase, which caused many young women to pop in on their way to work to get ready, and perhaps contributed partially to the unfeasibility of Biba's business model – the store closed less than two years after opening. The building still sells self-serve beauty, as a Marks & Spencer.

My other huge regret is that at age four, having decided to 'make my own perfume', I took the black art deco glass bottle of heady, patchouli-laced Biba cologne my mother had bought at Big Biba, and blended it with Christian Dior Eau Sauvage, Paco Rabanne and Chanel No 5 by pouring them all down the loo and stirring with a toilet brush. My mother caught me in the act and smacked me repeatedly on the backside, which, under the circumstances, I personally think rather restrained. I'd have killed me for a replacement.

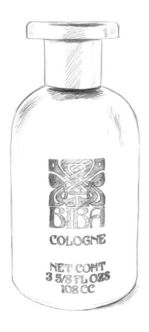

In a modern world of extreme contouring, it's hard to imagine that bronzer was ever not A Thing. Certainly, it wasn't commonly available in the eighties. The few bronzing powders on the high street were glittery, spangly affairs fit only for the disco. For make-up artists who wanted a flat, matte, not-too-orangey brown for lowlighting cheek hollows, narrowing noses, chiselling foreheads and generally warming pale-to-mid complexions, there was but one widely available product: Guerlain Terracotta Pour Homme.

This was a bronzing powder for men launched in 1984, at a time when male grooming was confined to two extremes: full-on New Romantic face painting or a macho routine of shower, sh*t, shave. It was unclear which of the two, if any, would accommodate a bronzer, and so I suspect the world's make-up artists alone kept Terracotta Pour Homme in production. The extraordinarily bulky, slightly odd domed packaging comprised a huge, stiff, wooden-topped, permanently overloaded brush that was utterly unusable for anyone not wanting to look like a tagine, but the pressed bronzer itself was glorious and indispensable on both men and women. Terracotta Pour Homme was used in every pop video (I'm prepared to put money on it being responsible for the razored cheekbones of the Robert Palmer 'Addicted to Love' girls), taken on every music tour, used on almost every photo shoot. The highly pigmented powder lasted for literally years of regular use (I still have mine from the eighties), which is perhaps where Guerlain came a cropper; they finally discontinued it a couple of years ago.

But feel no grief. Guerlain's Terracotta offering is now huge, unisex and contains an identically matte, velvety powder, minus the crazy brush, that is sleek enough to be transported without the aid of a roof-rack. And despite every brand in the world now making its own, Guerlain's is still arguably the best.

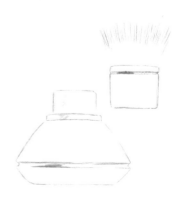

THE
GAME-
CHANGERS

There was a time when plucking one's brows meant dragging blunt, loose chemist tweezers across the skin, clasping desperately in the hope of pincering something, anything, then clumsily dragging it out before one had a chance to realise that this was an entirely crucial hair that solely represented the difference between stylish and startled. And so one rolled the dice again and again, picking away. It was a maddening process akin to defusing a bomb with a mohair knitting needle. I remember with horror my own first attempt at brow topiary, when I stood at a wall mirror and converted lush, dark brows into two toddler-drawn apostrophes, like Bette Davis as if stunned by police Taser.

Then came Tweezerman, the American tweezers imported by professional make-up artists before airlines outlawed them as hand luggage. Industry insiders and magazines positively raved about them but I couldn't begin to afford the £15 for my own (they were at least a tenner more than everyone else's) and so it was several years before my brows were treated with the respect they so critically deserve. By then I was a young journalist, unduly invited to Space NK's launch of their new brushes and tools collection. The store's then proprietor Nicky Kinnaird handed me my first pair of proper tweezers and declared these, not Tweezerman, to be the very best. It's fair to say that an hour later, in the loos of a posh London hotel, I experienced nothing short of a beauty epiphany. These were precision instruments that could as easily perform keyhole surgery as groom the brows of fidgety supermodels. The tiniest, seemingly inaccessible hairs were grasped with ease, then removed swiftly, elegantly and painlessly without gnawing off the surrounding area. The process was so unexpectedly gratifying that I immediately wanted to set up shop in the Ladies and pluck bald anyone passing through for a wee.

A little digging with the Space NK press office revealed that the manufacturer responsible was Rubis, a 60-year-old Swiss company specialising in the medical-grade tweezers used to assemble delicate Swiss clock and watch mechanics. Rubis's female founder had herself been frustrated with the atrocious quality of cosmetic tweezers and decided to apply her company's expertise to a retail product. Rubis now makes domestic tweezers under its own name, but also for Space NK, Bobbi Brown and a host of other luxury brands. Many remain devoted to their Tweezermans, and fair play to them. They are certainly decent. But my heart will always belong to Rubis, who, I believe, make the single best cosmetic tweezer the world has ever known. The Classic Slant is my weapon of choice for brow grooming, splinter removing, chin plucking (it genuinely makes the world's most depressingly middle-aged task a strangely gratifying one) and any other job for which I can conceivably deploy it. Trust me, it is well worth your cash.

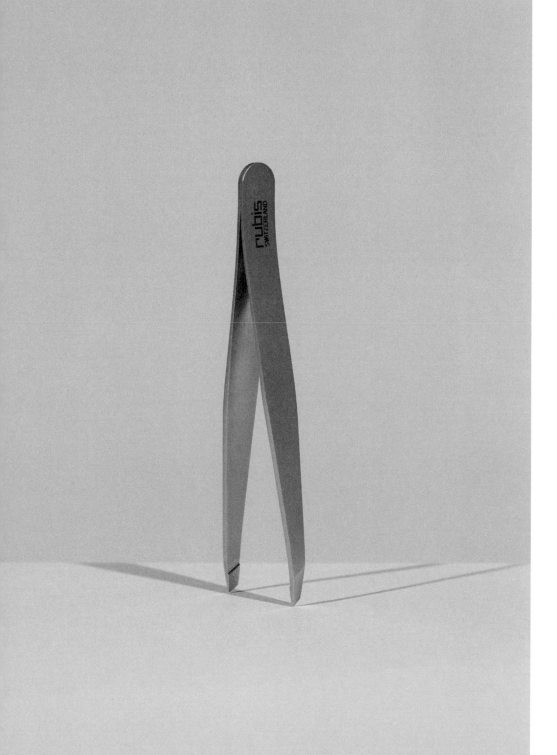

Blow drying is hard. I don't care who tells you otherwise, the average person cannot twist or oscillate a brush while simultaneously moving a dryer vertically downwards, all while seeing the world backwards in a mirror, any more than they can rub their tummies while patting their heads and performing a tap dance. We are just not wired this way, which is why there are now blow dry bars in every city, where it's basically impossible to get a last-minute appointment Wednesday through Saturday. Practicalities aside, few of us outside the Mayfair first wives club (they of huge unmovable hair and obnoxious chihuahua yapping from a Hermès Birkin) can afford to have our hair dried by a professional for anything but special occasions.

This is where the BaByliss Big Hair comes in. At first glance, it's a large, ugly lump of black plastic resembling a loo brush (which, while we're on the subject, should be banned) stuck to one of the Hoover tools whose purpose you never quite worked out. It comes in two sizes: large for long hair, medium for long bobs and above (this size is better if you have a fringe, too). In practice, this ingenious contraption (launched only in 2011) dries the hair while its brush-head twirls, just as your stylist would do with a separate dryer and barrel brush. If you overload the brush and your hair gets tangled, just hit the reverse button and the barrel will release it. It is, in my view, heaps faster if you blast your roots and hair with a classic dryer until it's about 80 per cent dry, then finish off with the Big Hair.

It would almost be perfect if it didn't ultimately give up the fight and slow to an unworkable speed. Mine have always done this after about eighteen months' use, but in all honesty I consider that pretty good in terms of cost-per-dry and a small price to pay for the kind of big, bouncy, straight hair previously beyond us civilians. In its own way, the Big Hair has changed my life and that of all my girlfriends. And for that reason, it is wholly deserving of the term gamechanger.

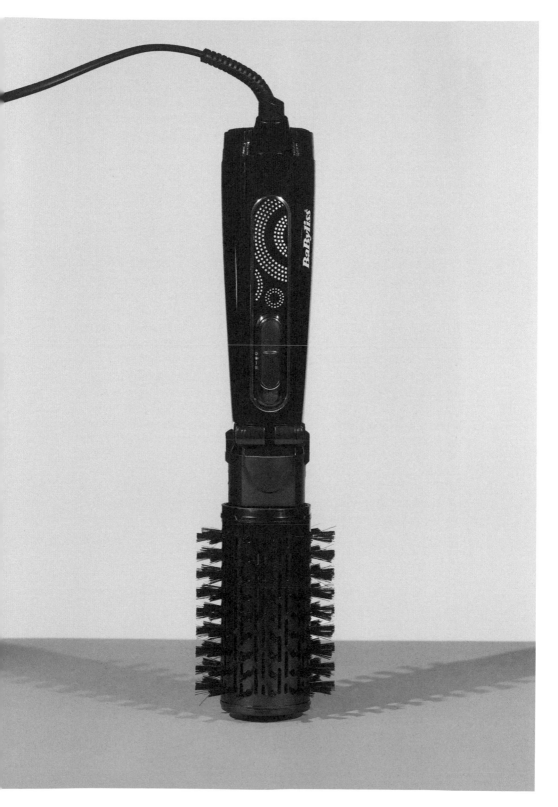

In the 1970s British people commonly had to wash their hair with the aid of a hot-cold-hot electric shower, plastic gravy jug or rubber shower hose attachment that pinged off at any pressure rise above dribble. Family holidays routinely consisted of grim communal shower blocks and endless queues of screaming kids and tutting campers. The launch of Batiste dry shampoo was an inspired solution, if a little grotty and hardly new in principle (women had been using talcum powder as an emergency scalp cleanser for decades). Batiste, a powdery, soapy-smelling hairspray, was to be applied to dry roots, left to absorb grease and general crap, then massaged and brushed through to remove chalky residue, in order to buy an extra day between proper shampoos. It was hugely useful for hospital stays and holidays but, somewhat reassuringly, remained a relatively unpopular substitute for real hair washing and went largely unnoticed next to the mosquito spray and car sickness tablets in the travel aisle of Boots.

But much in the same way that acne-zapping prescription retinoids were accidentally discovered to be the single best skin anti-ager we have, Batiste's true calling gradually emerged: 1990s hairdressers and punters observed that while it gave roots a 'whore's bath', Batiste was also visibly increasing volume and texture. Hair became thicker-looking, bigger, more able to hold style and shape. Ironically, clean locks lost their slip and acquired the matte finish of two-day-old hair, providing exactly the right grip for bridal tiaras, and kirbies in a beehive. Its instant volume acted as the perfect scaffolding for supermodel waves, big Hollywood barrel-curls and ratted rock-star tousles. Slowly, Batiste went from soap-dodging emergency measure to cult styling product, to mainstream beauty's go-to volumiser. It is now one of Britain's biggest selling hair products, owning almost 75 per cent of the huge dry shampoo market it spawned. A can of Batiste – now in countless fragrances, celebrity tie-in editions and packaging designs – is sold every two seconds in the UK alone and at time of writing, looks set to overtake the sales of proper wet-lather-rinse shampoo in some stores. Batiste is the *Shawshank Redemption* of beauty – a slow burner that eventually gained classic status.

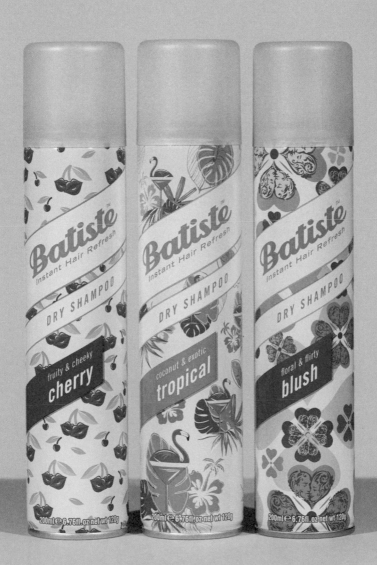

I have spent the last twenty years trying to love this product and I'm still not ready to let go. For me it's the make-up equivalent of *Modern Family*: I still don't get the appeal, but on I plough. My desperation stems from the fact that literally every make-up artist and beauty editor I know seems to love it, and much as I'm reliably obsessed with industry secrets and professional product recommendations in general, I think in this specific case that is exactly the problem. Secret Camouflage – a compact containing two complementary shades of waxy, full coverage concealer – is, for me, a brilliant and essential product for anyone who makes up multiple faces on a regular basis. One of each Secret Camouflage colourway will guarantee a match with practically any skin, from snow white to espresso black, because any of the shades can be mixed with another to darken, lighten or warm.

The problem for me is in consumer use. Unless you are in and out of the sun with no SPF (I daren't even go there), your skin will basically always be the same colour, which rather begs the question of why you'd want to mix your own base every day, when you could just buy a single concealer in the right colour from the get-go. A single concealer is faster, more convenient to use and consistent in tone, and doesn't require an extra brush. There is, I suppose, an argument that tone varies from area to area – under eyes are bound to have more blue or grey tones than the chin, for example – and so a different concealer may be needed. But I don't find either of the tones in Secret Camouflage to be sufficiently bold as to correct serious discolouration (and why should it? It's a concealer, not a corrector), and I simply can't be bothered with the faff of mixing up different tones, and so I'd rather use two separate products.

My other issue is one of waste, something that pains me in any aspect of beauty (and life). Whenever I trawl through a make-up bag containing Secret Camouflage (remarkably often), I know before I've even popped the compact that I'll find one colour down to the metal pan and the other at best almost full, at worst barely smeared. I find the idea of paying top dollar to use half a product fairly intolerable.

But what I will certainly concede is that Secret Camouflage was a gamechanger, and has been hugely influential on the industry as a whole. It was among the first products to encourage women to be their own make-up artists, creating bespoke shades, considering undertones and employing professional techniques, particularly in Mercier's specialist area of skin. The formula itself is very good – creamy but unmovable, densely pigmented without blotchiness. It also deserves to be classed as an icon, since, if I found it missing from a professional kit, I would possibly die of shock.

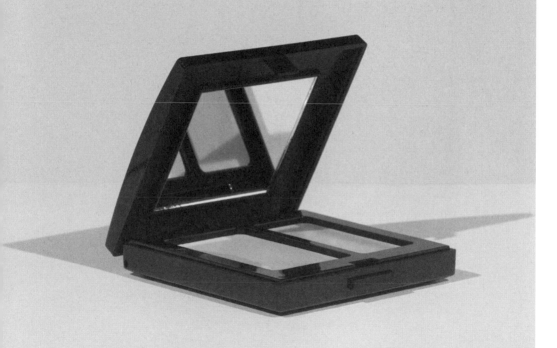

The nerdy story behind the Astalift brand – the first cosmetic project from Fuji, the photographic company – immediately got my attention at its 2011 launch. Fuji had wondered if the antioxidants and collagen used in colour film to stop photographs fading could be adapted for skincare use. It was sitting on exclusive, patented camera film technology that allowed it to come up with tinier microparticles of collagen than had ever before been used in skincare, thus allowing the ingredient to be better, and more deeply absorbed into the skin – or so the theory went.

I was particularly intrigued by Astalift's hero product, Jelly Aquarysta, a decidedly weird-looking red gel-serum in a frankly naff-looking red and gold pot like something from the Poundshop (incidentally, why, oh why do beauty companies spend so much on research, development and patenting, only to then insist on packaging antioxidants and other delicate ingredients in jars and pots where they are soon destabilised and made less effective? It infuriates me. Airtight pumps, please. It's not the fifties). There were no clinical trials available to me at the time and so I was sceptical, but the uniqueness of the product – wobbly and bright red, like something one might scrape off a trestle table at the end of a toddler's birthday party – made me get it out of the cupboard and take it for a spin. I took a pea-sized amount and massaged it in after cleansing and before moisturising, morning and night. At bedtime, I added serum over the top of the super-fine-textured jelly, too.

The results were remarkable. Where my face, having undergone a brutal few months of hard work and late nights, had been looking grey, dull and thin, it now appeared clearer, brighter, plumper and more even. The skin around my eyes was noticeably smoother. The gel was absorbed immediately into the skin with absolutely no grease, making it suitable for all skins, even oily. Make-up glided beautifully over the top. People kept telling me I looked well when they weren't after something. I positively raved about the product like someone fresh from an Alpha Course, and, so great is my power and influence over British consumer habits, that Astalift responded by almost immediately withdrawing from the market. You can still buy Astalift outside Britain and, to be perfectly honest, it's still pretty easy to buy online here, but I do fear for its future in the longer term. My advice, should you see it marked down in T.K. Maxx, as many of my readers have, is to pick some up.

It can be quite cheering to find a practice in modern life that technology has failed to transform. Copper razors first appeared some 5,000 years ago, and despite the advent of electric devices as far back as the early 1930s, the good old-fashioned wet shave is still the preferred method of the hairless majority. The principle of the razor hasn't changed all that much in five millennia, though of course the equipment has developed a tiny bit since Adam hit puberty, or we'd still be plucking out hairs with pairs of shells. Since the appearance of the safety razor in the nineteenth century, advances in design have chiefly concerned either convenience of use or quality of shave.

Gillette introduced a two-blade razor as early as 1971, and added a lubricating strip soon afterwards. Next came a pivoting head, and in 1990 the Gillette Sensor made its debut. The Sensor's great leap forward was to individually spring-load the blades so that the razor responded to the curves of the user's face. Face, not legs or underarms, as this was no unisex razor – the musclebound TV commercials and 'The best a man can get' tagline couldn't be much less ambiguous. Except that for me, and every other woman I knew, the Sensor was when razors stopped being crap. The Sensor navigated knees, ankles and underarms without nick, scrape or rash. Having tried our dads' or boyfriends' for size, we couldn't get our own fast enough.

In fairness, Gillette isn't a company that can be accused of neglecting female customers. In fact it launched the first razor for women, the unimprovably named Milady Décolleté, in 1915. Here, Gillette didn't just cater to a market, but arguably created one. Aimed at 'the modern woman who would appear at her best – who cares for those little niceties of habit', it put the very notion of shaved pits into the minds of a generation of women, to many of whom underarm hair had been, up to that point, a non-issue. One could argue that Gillette created a problem for women, purely so that it could fix it for a price.

Sensor for Women followed its masculine counterpart in 1992, replacing the black and silver tubular design of the male version with a wide flat unit of white plastic surrounding a turquoise central panel, ridged for better grip. The responsiveness of the springs made shaving previously hazardous contours a pleasure; this seemingly modest technological advance actually proved far more of a tangible improvement to the shaving experience than Gillette's subsequent (and alarmingly expensive) multi-blade obsession – three on the Mach3/Venus in 1998, five on 2006's Fusion (with a sixth 'precision' blade on the back) and presumably a hundred by the time they launch the Gillette Centurion in 2035.

It was almost inevitable that after several years of men and women straightening their hair flat with irons and dousing them in serum until they resembled Crufts-ready Afghans (I'm ashamed to include myself in that), we'd crave a counterpoint. Then came young actress Sienna Miller with her tasselled sandals and boho cheesecloth skirts (shudder) and with them, soft, surfer girl waves that whispered 'effortless' while being almost impossible for any layperson to achieve. On shoots, meanwhile, professional stylists had taken to hot-tonging straight hair into haphazard waves, then using spray bottles filled with real saltwater to create tousles and rough, matte texture.

Since landlocked women were unlikely to travel to the coast for a good hair day (I'm ashamed to exclude myself from that), nor enjoy the drying effect of regular saltwater styling, cool New York hair salon Bumble and Bumble wisely developed Surf Spray. This is a unisex product containing real sea kelp and added moisturisers, that when sprayed into damp hair before air or rough drying gives straight, floppy-type locks just enough grit to hold mermaid waves and just enough sea-swept messiness to make the wearer appear to give not too much of a damn (it even *smells* like the sea). Surf Spray was an instant hit, appearing in what seemed like every summer beauty shoot and cool celebrity get-the-look page for years on end. I cannot think of a single product that so completely defined a moment in beauty and yet so enduringly influenced the entire industry in the process.

Casual, unkempt hair has remained a key trend ever since (I'm still unfailingly asked how to achieve beach waves at reader events), with only scant evolution. There are now many copycats – from high end to high street – and Bumble themselves have built on Surf Spray's enormous success with a 'Surf' shampoo, conditioner, infusion (Surf Spray for dry, thick hair types, essentially) and mousse, but the original remains the King of the Waves. A word of caution seems fair: Surf Spray looks fabulously beachy on day one. Apply again on day two and hair looks as though it hasn't been near any water, never mind the ocean, in at least six months.

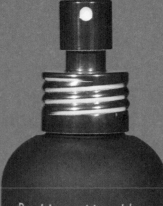

It's perhaps hard to imagine now, but when I entered the beauty industry in 1990 most foundations were for Caucasian women with skin the colour of candy floss. Seriously, almost everything available in the shops had unfathomably pink undertones that made white skin look sickly, while brown and black skins were almost wholly uncatered for outside 'specialist' brands. Professional make-up artists would either mix in a dollop of pure banana-yellow pigment or go to pro stores for a small, extremely expensive cult range called Visiora by Christian Dior. It seems so strange that a mainstream consumer beauty industry made only foundations for the 10 or so per cent of women who needed a pink base (Celtic-type skin tones, generally), and ignored the indisputable truth that most skins look prettiest when bathed in yellow light, like candleglow.

In 1992 a New York make-up artist called Bobbi Brown took matters into her own hands. Off the back of the success of her small, sell-out range of neutral-toned lipsticks, Brown launched Foundation Stick, a range of flatteringly yellow-toned bases for women of all ethnicities. The portable, solid formulation, made spreadable by the warmth of the skin, allowed finger, brush or sponge application either all over the face or in smaller areas in need of coverage. Coverage was buildable, from sheer to full, never heavy or caked. Pink could be added separately as a corrector, to lighten under-eye dark circles or brighten any dullness, leaving the rest of the face soft and natural-looking ('yellow' foundations in the right shade don't make skin look yellow, they just make it look like skin). Brown has since launched over a dozen different foundations, from tinted moisturisers and oil-free liquid to tinted serums and solid compacts, but Foundation Stick remains her bestseller (one is sold every minute globally).

One subtle reformulation aside (the modern version is more hydrating and easier to work with), this hero base remains as brilliant as ever, and without question influenced the now widespread production of yellow tones across the entire beauty market. Bobbi Brown's commitment to accessible, multiracial beauty also proved groundbreaking. A woman of any hue or age can visit a Bobbi Brown counter and leave with everything she needs to look fantastic. Few other mainstream brands – MAC is one, perhaps also Estée Lauder nowadays – can make this boast, and while we perhaps shouldn't be so pathetically grateful to see vast groups of women acknowledged by big business, we should value its fundamental human decency nonetheless. I always keep a Foundation Stick in my make-up bag (despite my perfect shade, Cool Beige, being discontinued) because its non-spill, non-breakable metal tube makes it endlessly practical for mid-afternoon touch-ups, weekends away and for taking on romantic dates that may just result in a sleepover.

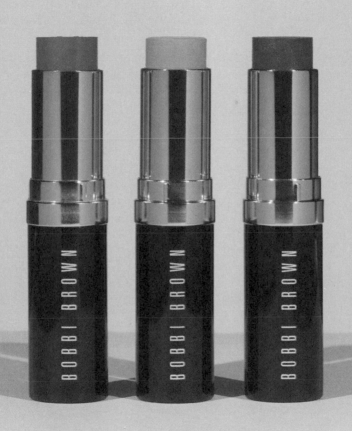

I can honestly say that I have not been on a single photo shoot in the last decade and not seen this product, lid flipped up, ready for action or newly used, at the make-up artist's workstation. There it remained for years until an explosion in French pharmacy brands in around 2013. Bioderma, along with Vichy, Roc and Embryolisse, is a mid-price (known in the business by the quite awful portmanteau of 'masstige' – as in mass market and prestige) brand loved by beauty editors and make-up artists who routinely stocked up almost as soon as Louboutin touched chaussée outside the Gare du Nord.

Sensing its products might travel, Bioderma began exporting its hero, Créaline make-up remover, to Britain's beauty professional stores. The press went crazy, stocks flew, and so the rest of the range soon followed its trail. Most of the Bioderma range – now available nationwide at Boots – is solid, but Créaline (now renamed Sensibio H2O) is special because it introduced an entirely new category in beauty to non-French consumers. It's a 'micellar water', a clear, non-rinse cleanser containing micelles – tiny round balls of cleansing molecules suspended in water. Like all micellars, Créaline is swept over skin with a cotton wool pad, and the micelles cling to dirt and make-up, removing them swiftly and effectively.

This fast, extremely gentle way of cleansing makes micellar perfect for speedy backstage make-up changeovers at fashion shows and photo shoots (when model skin may well have already taken a battering), and particularly convenient for use by normal women who might be staying in hospital, camping or flying, or those who are too tired, weak or sloshed to engage in the rigmarole of proper hot cloth cleansing at a sink. It's marvellous for skins easily aggravated by beauty products and endlessly useful for everyone else. Love Créaline though I do (particularly in this, its Hydrabio H2O incarnation – an extra hydrating version with a blue label), it is not, in my view, a long-term substitute for thorough cleansing with a balm or oil and flannel. It's better than wipes, certainly, but over time will not keep skin looking its very best. It can, in some cases (including my own), even cause spots. But as a short term emergency solution, it's unbeatable.

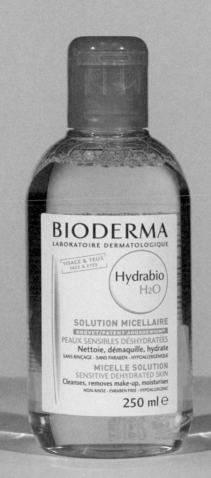

'Forget those plugs and cords, girls, you don't need them no more . . .': so went the jingle for Braun Independent, the revolutionary cordless hair styler for busy women on the move. This was a handbag-friendly hot brush that transformed into a curling tong, powered by replaceable butane gas canisters sold in supermarkets and chemists. I can still hear the click-click-click of the Braun's ignition, followed by the hiss of the gas heating up the chamber, turning the little red indicator sticker to black. The Braun Independent caused something of a scandal within weeks of its launch, when British school kids realised they could huff the fuel canisters behind the geography prefab to get high, and very possibly die in the process. Braun hastily designed safer, sealed gas cartridges, but the by now school-wide ban only increased the gadget's desirability. Everyone wanted a Braun Independent, not least because they were exactly the right tool for shaping your 1980s demiwave or taming your shaggy perm, all while inwardly screaming, 'I'm a modern woman who might stay out all night! I have no time for my mum's plug-in Carmens!'

That said, my working mother was such a devotee of the Braun Independent that her green Austin Mini was littered with its mismatched component parts and half-empty gas canisters that could easily have gone mushroom cloud whenever she sparked up a Silk Cut. We were once approached, amid a chorus of horn beeping, by a Gwent police officer wanting to know why she was curling her hair in the rear-view mirror instead of moving on at a green light. Truly, this was post-modern feminism in action.

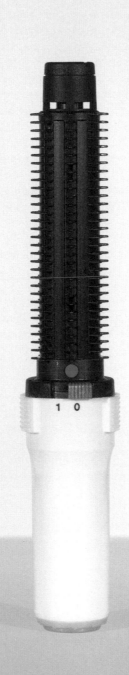

The Caucasian male grooming regime moves from one decade to another with essentially little change. Hair slightly longer, hair trimmed shorter, the odd beard trend or foray into poodle perms – this woeful lack of options is one of the many reasons not to want to be a man, and, for me at least, just about negates their ability to stand and pee into a hedge. Revolutions are rare, but this fat, Pritt-stick-style hair wax certainly helped one gather momentum. For years on end, men's hair was either untouched by product or positively smothered in wet-look hair gel or cream to flatten or corral it into retro quiffs or mean spikes. It gave the impression that hair was there to be tamed, greased or gunked into submission, as though it were nothing more than a nuisance or obstacle.

Then, in the nineties, men's hair fought back. Matte waxes (as opposed to the shiny pomade versions like Black & White and Dax Wax) came onto the market, and could be used to lift and shape hair with minimal faff and plenty of texture. Ironically, it was a product that could be worked through the hair to make it look less done, more effortless and natural, a little bit, well, *shagged*. At the beginning of this new wax trend, Anthony Mascolo, session stylist and Creative Director at Toni & Guy salons, was using so much matte wax on clients and male models that his hands were permanently gross, and he realised that application direct from a stick, much like a giant lipstick, would suit him and his clients a bit better.

The resulting Bed Head Wax Stick was as instant a success as any product I've ever known. Truly, it seemed like overnight every cool boy had one in his bathroom, every male Britpop artist bore the hallmarks of a good going over with Bed Head (though I'm not naive enough to think sex, booze, weed and cocaine didn't heighten the overall effect of dishevelment). I'd pass matted, shaggy indie haircuts in the street and know Bed Head was responsible, and be hit by the (very pleasant) Bed Head smell every time I entered a decent bar or club. It was the first time in ages that a cool grooming product had been made exclusively for men to enjoy without it having to justify its existence with macho slogans and packaging like engine oil. Looking after one's appearance was no longer a chore, an embarrassment or best left to the girls, it was a pleasure in itself. Bed Head was trendy, covetable, influential and, I think, rang the starting bell on modern male grooming.

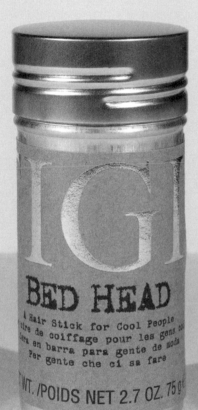

A pot containing a hollow sponge, soaked with nail polish remover, in which to poke a painted nail for just a second, before pulling out of the well, clean as a whistle. Such an ingenious idea for travel and a simple solution to the problem of finding cotton wool and disposing of it afterwards without stinking out the house. I couldn't live without it, I admire it, I take it on every holiday, every photo shoot, and recommend it widely.

But, it must be said, Bourjois didn't invent it. Pretty Quik, at half the price and working on the exact same principle, came first and for years I thought I was the only one who'd heard of it, until I began working at *ELLEgirl* magazine and smelled Pretty Quik's unmistakable fumes wafting from the desk of a staff writer. Lucy always kept Pretty Quik in her pedestal for quick nail changes before after-work drinks and so we'd frequently set up nail shop in the features department. It wasn't for another ten years, in 2012, that Bourjois, perhaps unwittingly, got the same idea and it finally caught on. Now there are several versions. Leighton Denny, Ciaté and Nails Inc all released their own take on the Pretty Quik concept but, on balance, Bourjois (the first of the new crop) seems to have the best sponge, smell, packaging and speed.

And so, while Bourjois were not the innovators here, they were the gamechangers, in that they finally got everyone to notice what is an utterly brilliant invention. There's now a 2-in-1 version, with the addition of a sponge in the lid for removing toe polish (very much Bourjois's concept), but I confess to being somewhat skeeved by the idea of a toe sponge festering inside a pot for weeks on end, however steeped in chemicals. For me, the joy of the magic finger pot is in its simplicity. It is a perfect beauty problem solver and there's no need to gild the lily.

Writer Nora Ephron claimed repeatedly that the reason mature women look younger than ever isn't related to feminism, exercise, health or even to plastic surgery. It's all about hair dye. And as much as it pains me to say it, as a person who can no longer safely cover greys due to a severe late-onset allergy to PPD (the ingredient in almost all dyes), Ephron was characteristically on the money. I firmly believe that teeth and hair determine how old we look, much less so wrinkles. And while there's nothing wrong with leaving your hair to grey naturally – on the contrary, a head of silver is fabulously chic – around two-thirds of us ultimately reach for the bottle, and why not? Other than that dyeing is a time-consuming and expensive business. I know several women who have to ringfence two hours of their time and at least fifty quid of their hard-earned cash each and every month, in order to visit a salon for a root tint.

My advice is always that they should buy this, an ingenious little kit that, quite unfathomably, blends greys with literally any shade of blonde, brown, red and black, despite only coming in fourteen colourways. You must always patch test for allergies first, of course. After that, the technique is so easy and straightforward that you can quite conceivably dye your hair before work in ten minutes flat. Just mix together the little bottle of chemicals and tube of colourant in the dinky tray provided, part your dry hair in the normal way, and brush on the dye. Wait ten minutes, rinse. That's it. No stained towels, no shower caps, no squirty bottles, no panicking that you've missed a bit, no greys. To describe Root Touch-Up further would be to do it a disservice. It is beyond simple, completely genius and should easily buy you a couple of extra weeks between appointments, which may well change your life. My great sadness is that I can no longer use it.

For many women, myself included, there was life before GHD and then there was life after it. Life BGHD, pre-2001, consisted of big, clunky metal hair straighteners like portable sandwich toasters on a stick. They took an age to heat and use, with the irons having to be dragged through the same section repeatedly before it would lie almost flat. This ritual abuse caused dryness, breakage and split ends and attempts to minimise damage with gimmicky add-ons like steaming water cartridges attached to the plates, much like on a household iron, failed to make straighteners any more pleasant to use. This was manageable, if wearisome, until fashion hurtled towards super-straight, sleek locks like a show pony's mane.

Like everything else in 2001, it was all about Rachel from *Friends*. After growing out the original 'Rachel' cut, a multi-layered, big, pouffy, long bob that had sent the world into a copycat frenzy, actress Jennifer Aniston and her now famous hairdresser Chris McMillan had distanced themselves by making Rachel's new hair as flat, silky and sleek as possible. Celebrities took Aniston's lead and straight hair became the ideal hairstyle for women everywhere. By the time we reached *Friends*' season 7 in 2001, Rachel's hair was a blunt-cut bob with flicky-out ends that couldn't hope to be achieved without either a professional or a dramatically better home hair tool.

Two British entrepreneurs and a hairstylist travelled to Korea to find a solution and discovered a prototype for a new kind of straightener, using ceramic, rather than metal, plates. Traditional straighteners had heated hair from the outside in, scorching the surface, causing damage and frizz. The heat from ceramics worked faster, penetrating hair quickly, heating it evenly from inside out. They heated to a high temperature within a minute or so, straightened hair more uniformly and much more thoroughly, in a fraction of the time, causing less damage in the process. The irons themselves were thin, allowing them to reach the root of the hair and be used for precision styling of small sections like spikes, flicks and fringes. The trio bought the worldwide rights, set up business in Leeds, and the GHD (an acronym for Good Hair Day) Styler, costing four times as much as those we'd used previously, was born.

I have never known such an expensive beauty product become so ubiquitous in such a short space of time – much less one that neither advertised nor sold in high street retailers. Within the best part of a year, GHD was no longer a hair tool, it was a verb: 'I've just ghd'd my hair.' Every hairdresser used the styler, Madonna and Gwyneth Paltrow each owned a set. Naturally, Jennifer Aniston swore by hers, and even when she, Rachel and their fans moved on to a more textured, casual look, GHD was ready for the shift, promoting ways of using the original styler to create curls, waves and flicks, attracting a male clientele in the process. Nowadays, instant heat, digital control, thin plates (whether made of ceramic, titanium or tourmaline) are standard across all quality straighteners, and, sadly, we expect to pay the best part of £100 to own them.

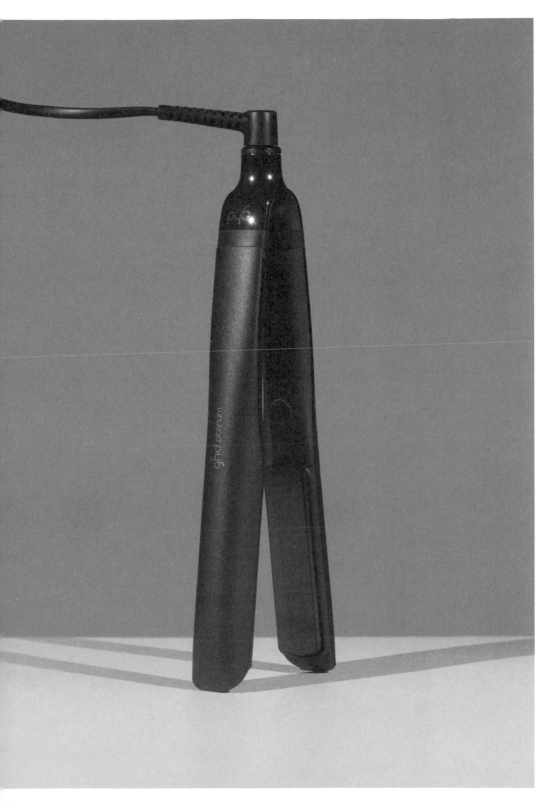

Are you a smudger? Because I bet I can still out-smudge you. Put any traditional mascara on my puny lashes, however carefully and patiently, and I guarantee that within the hour I'll have black, gritty under-eye stains like the tracks of a bicycle wheel on a rainy day. This is, I came to realise many years ago, in no small part thanks to my dry skin and its need for rich, heavy under-eye moisturiser that lifts mascara from its station – though oily types and hormonal hot flashers may find their skin's natural lubricants do the same. For the first half of my adult life, my only way to avoid panda eyes was to forgo the emollients and enjoy uncomfortable, flaky skin instead.

Until one day in late 2002, when I took a meeting with a representative from Covent Garden independent beauty boutique Pout. I was given a tiny anonymous-looking tube of mascara called Blinc, and an evangelical sales pitch promising it wouldn't budge. Pfft. I tried it more out of sheer bloody-mindedness than any belief it might actually work. But it did. Here was a mascara that stayed on with no flakes, smudges, runs, itching or irritation, developed in response to company owner Lewis Farsedakis hearing his fiancée complain about all five. The secret was in his radically different formula, made from liquid polymers instead of the traditional oils, waxes, fibres and dye. The plasticky, wet-looking liquid wrapped itself around each lash as it dried, lengthening and slightly thickening it with a flexible tube of dense black mascara. Unlike traditional mascaras that were removed either deliberately or by rain, sweat and oil, this had to be sodden with warm water, causing the tubes to expand and slip off. My obsession with this new technology led me to Kevyn Aucoin, who had built on the tubing concept with Japanese chemists to introduce his own curling and volumising versions of Blinc's orginal, and Eyeko, early adopters of Blinc's technique.

Gradually, as years passed and word of mouth spread, the mass-market brands pricked up their ears. Now, while still dwarfed in numbers by traditional formulas, tubing mascaras appear on every high street. Estée Lauder Double Wear, Clinique Lash Power, MAC Opulash, Too Faced Lash Injection and Djv-beautenizer Fiberwig are just some of the best, but it should be noted that no mascara gives the dramatic, thick, falsies (and in my case, smudged to hell) effect of a traditional fibre mascara. And so where massive, fluttery lashes are required, I suggest applying an old-school mascara first, then locking the whole thing down with a tubing formula. I've done it for years and it works a treat.

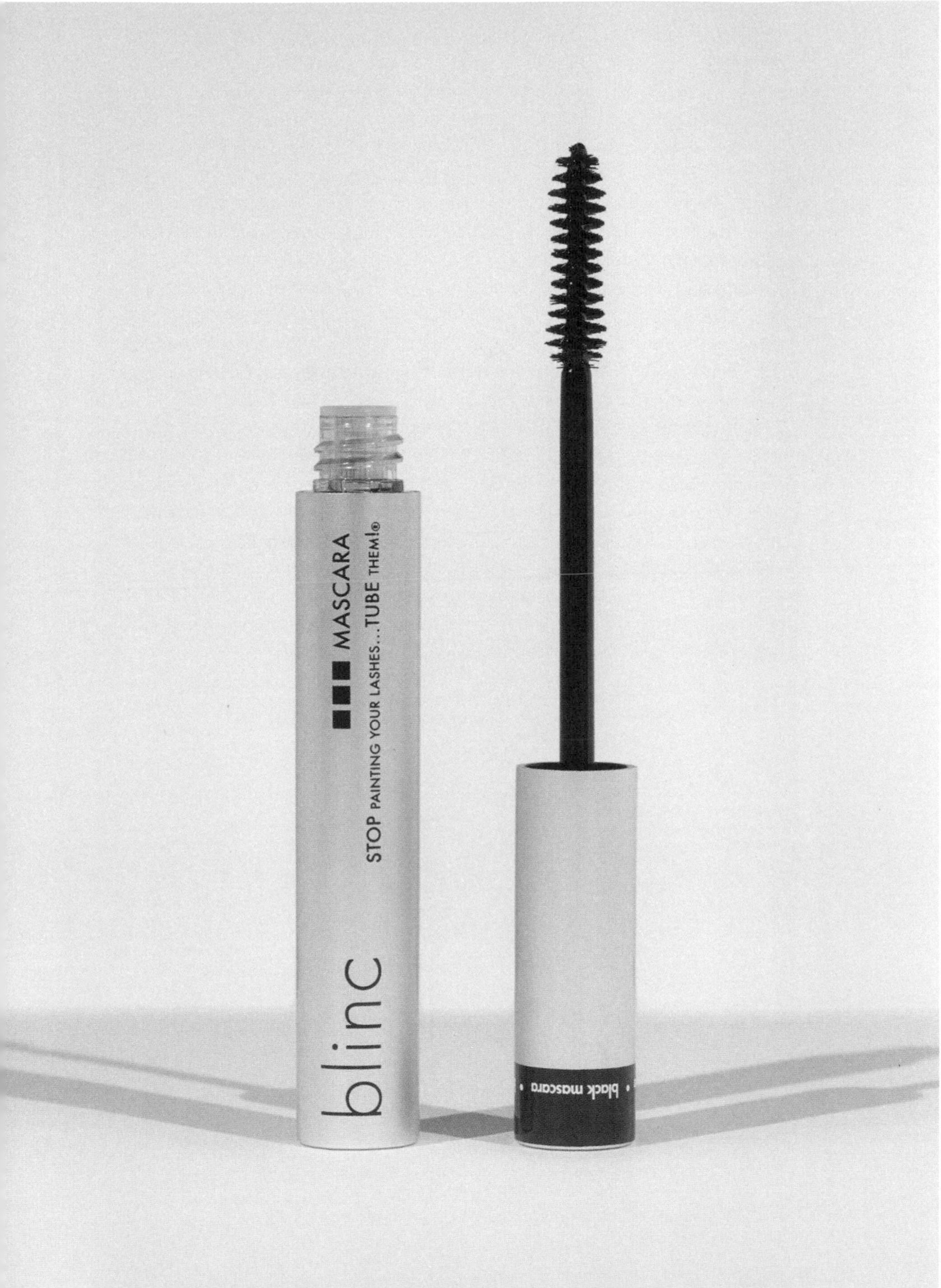
blinc
MASCARA
STOP PAINTING YOUR LASHES... TUBE THEM!®
black mascara

Clinique Suncare

There is absolutely no question that Clinique suncare products are of great quality. They're reliable, kind to skin, neither peel under make-up nor make my eyes stream. But they're not unique in any of those areas. Where Clinique suncare changed the game was in its self-imposed ban on any sun protection factor below 15. This was a radical decision in the mid-eighties, when a significant number of customers were happy to baste themselves in factor 4 or 8 and kid themselves they'd emerge looking like Gisele rolled in molasses. In fact, they were potentially doing themselves grave harm. Dermatologists are in broad agreement that any SPF below 15 is barely worth a damn in reducing the risk of sun damage, while research shows SPF15 protects against 93 per cent of UVB radiation. Personally, I'm a 30 on my body, a 50 on my face – at least in summer months – but I also live at the seaside and have seen enough blistered chests and peeling noses to know that an industry shift towards factor 15 represents a stride in the right direction.

A couple of years after the Clinique initiative, its parent company, Estée Lauder, also made the then bold decision to sell only broad-spectrum sunscreens across all its brands; that is, protection against both UVB rays (those most likely to burn the skin, the protection from which is a legal requirement in UK sunscreens) and UVA (those most likely to age the skin, the protection from which, in the eyes of the law, is an optional extra). If only both, or even either, of these initiatives were catching – there are still plenty of brands, at all price points from bargain to luxury, putting profits before public protection. I wish them a million cloudy days.

People often forget about Elizabeth Arden, one of the founding mothers of modern beauty, but the brand is more than a heritage house – it still carries some of the most cleverly formulated make-up staples a woman can buy. They're just frustratingly well hidden. These genius eye pencils are my all-time favourites. They are, quite simply, the easiest, fastest route to the smoky look most women seem to feel is beyond them. Developed in 1996 when make-up artist Mary Greenwell was creative consultant, they look like any other pencil, but the 'lead', instead of being made from wax, is actually a tightly pressed powder. This combines the best of both worlds: the precision, control and convenience of a pencil and the soft, forgiving blendability of an eyeshadow. And so the pencils – in black, a lovely gunmetal grey and, my favourite, espresso brown – can be stroked along the lashline (and inside it, for a truly authentic smoky eye) in a fairly haphazard fashion, then just smudged with the sponge at the end of the pencil to give a professional-looking, rather sexy, line.

They may not be famous themselves (and I really will never understand why Elizabeth Arden essentially behaves as though they don't exist), but Smoky Eyes Pencils have certainly inspired many others. Charlotte Tilbury's wonderful Classic Pencil is a dead ringer, for example. Estée Lauder's Magic Smoky Powder crayons have the same idea, though are a bit too fat to be as useful. But however many I've loved, I always return to the original and become quite anxious as I run out. It's frustratingly hard to find Arden now; its department store presence is greatly diminished in no small part owing, I suspect, to the brand's rather muddled product line and counter environment in recent times. But things are improving steadily and its recent acquisition by Revlon is, I think, promising. Unlike some huge, soulless takeover by a detergent or pharma corporation, this deal represents the union of two old-school beauty legends. I am hopeful for a return to glory.

Pre-1979, deep conditioner was, at least to white women, a treatment their hairdresser might talk them into to make an extra few quid on an appointment. A salon-only product was painted on or massaged into broken, dry, chemically overdosed hair, wrapped and placed under a dryer to soften, temporarily seal and add gloss. Not that there weren't any DIY methods of taking extra care of hair. One might leave in regular conditioner overnight, massage in some oil, whether of the bath or cooking variety (it's absolutely true that when I was a little girl, olive oil came from the chemist, not the supermarket), or, notably, VO5 Hot Oil, a little tube to be dropped into a cup of hot water to warm before application, launched by Alberto-Culver to considerable success three years previously. But deep conditioners as we know them, or as a beauty category in their own right, didn't really exist and certainly the haircare industry hadn't yet caught up with the 1970s home hairstyling revolution and the dryness and damage caused by its heated rollers and crimping irons.

At this time, American Tom Redmond Snr, a somewhat eccentric entrepreneur already working in the hair salon industry, was travelling through the Australian bush when he met a chemist who'd developed a 'hair reconstructing potion' (how very scientific) from thirty-six moisturising and nourishing ingredients, many of them – like aloe, sea kelp and custard apple – originating in Oz. He shipped it home, named it Aussie 3 Minute Miracle, quit his job, and, along with his chemist, set about expanding the Aussie range to include shampoos, regular conditioner and styling. But it was 3 Minute Miracle that caused the stir. Via rave reviews and word of mouth, women bought into the novelty of both deep conditioner and its provenance (like footwear company Ugg, Aussie haircare celebrates and capitalises on the antipodean origins of its product, while being about as Australian as the Pentagon), and soon the rest of the market followed suit.

Personally, I find 3 Minute Miracle too heavy for my fine hair (I do, however, love the Aussie 2-in-1 Aussome Volume, an unusually good combined shampoo and conditioner). Natural-haired women of colour will find it too light, curly girls may be put off by the inclusion of silicone (the ingredients have changed several times since the trip to the Australian bush), many may find its strong, fruity scent a bit like showering in Haribo Starmix. But countless women with dry, permed, relaxed or coloured hair are absolutely evangelical about this product, claiming it softens, moisturises, defrizzes and conditions better than anything and won't countenance the use of another deep conditioner. There are now several conditioners in the Mega Moisture franchise, selling almost 3.2 million bottles a year in the UK, but the original Reconstructor still dominates with over a third of the share. The Redmond family have long since cashed out but their baby remains, by some distance, Britain's bestselling hair treatment.

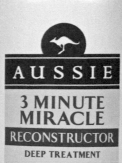

AUSSIE

3 MINUTE MIRACLE

RECONSTRUCTOR

DEEP TREATMENT

for damaged hair

with **Australian Balm Mint** extract
Our special formula with **Australian Balm Mint** extract smoothes rough cuticles and helps restore manageability and adds shine.

MANAGEABILITY & SHINE

250 ml e

Calvin Klein's CK One turned apathy into an art form. Launched with Steven Meisel's arresting shots of a waifish, 20-year-old Kate Moss and assorted beautiful young things, CK One instantly made any pushy beauty campaign fronted by a buxom, varnished supermodel seem terribly old hat. Abetted by cultural markers like *Trainspotting* and the deaths of River Phoenix and Kurt Cobain, the fragrance's groundbreaking campaigns helped push 'heroin chic' firmly into the mid-nineties zeitgeist. CK One couldn't be bothered. The models couldn't be bothered to seek your patronage. The ads couldn't be bothered to be in colour. Moss couldn't be bothered to deliver the tagline to the TV commercial with any more enthusiasm than a schoolgirl forced by a history teacher to read out an intercepted note.

But the insouciance of the delivery (which echoes down the years in countless languid, barely audible fragrance ad payoffs) shouldn't distract from the significance of the message: 'A fragrance for a man or a woman'. CK One was not the first unisex fragrance, but it was the first to market itself so distinctly as such, and with phenomenal success: at its peak, selling twenty bottles a minute and annually turning over in the region of $90 million. In keeping with the brand's general air of indifference and the requirements of a true unisex scent, the fragrance itself – latterly promoted by a new generation of unbothered teens in 2014's twentieth anniversary campaign – evidences no overbearing personality. A good, clean, citrus, 'straight out of the shower' scent, CK One is just the androgynous shrug its marketing implied. It couldn't be bothered to be anything else.

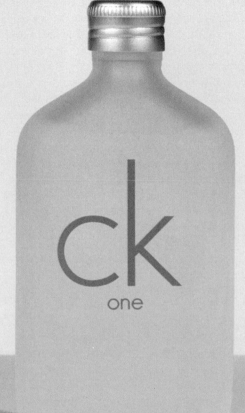

Every few months or so, I read a piece on how bespoke-mixed beauty products are the next big thing and think again how utterly, and unluckily, ahead of its time Prescriptives was. Born into the Estée Lauder companies in 1979, Prescriptives was a science-driven brand for women of all ethnicities, who struggled to find make-up to match their skin's tone and type. It catered for them all in two revolutionary ways. The brand created an extremely wide spectrum of foundation shades and formulations (over a hundred at one point), each of them available in a variety of undertones and coded accordingly – Yellow/Orange for warm, golden undertones, Red/Orange for peach undertones, Red for cool pink, Blue/Red for cool rose – much as MAC does now with its C, N, NC and NW base coding. At Prescriptives these were identified in a customer's skin with the use of an on-counter colour wheel, narrowing down the entire Prescriptives offering to flattering, complementary shades. On the slim chance a customer couldn't be matched from stock, a consultant could mix a Custom Blend foundation and powder, B&Q Dulux paint machine-style, adding extra coverage, colour correctors and skin treatments to the mix. Individual recipes were then stored on file for repeat purchases.

It has to be said that Prescriptives' counters, while offering a skilled and important service, were not a laugh-a-minute. I always felt beauty was presented as a problem to fix, rather than a pleasure in itself. The packaging was uninspiring and self-consciously serious. Compacts and bottle caps were made from the sort of depressing grey plastic normally reserved for Job Club stacking chairs or the office wastepaper bin. But the product within was extraordinarily good. Magic Liquid Potion and Powder (inspired by film special effect make-up) were an instant, camera-ready complexion perfector and retouching powder respectively, on sale a decade before Instagram was ever invented, and are exactly the kind of product that now lands on my desk on a weekly basis, claiming to be groundbreaking. Virtual Skin was among the first really natural-looking foundations available, while Exact Match, the first foundation I ever worked with as a make-up assistant, was the first to tweak ingredients purely to ensure women of colour didn't get an ashy complexion.

As the rest of the industry caught up with Prescriptives' colour matching philosophy and did so with a little more joy and luxury, Prescriptives struggled to hold on. In 2009 Estée Lauder spiked the brand, declaring its future untenable. Prescriptives customers had other ideas. Two years and 25,000 emails later, the brand returned online only, selling its most popular products and making up new batches of their US customers' individual custom blend recipes. At time of writing, international shipping is unavailable. British women can seek consolation only in the fact that Prescriptives' deservedly beloved fresh, melony perfume, Calyx, has been adopted by the Clinique family and is available at their counters nationwide.

I like to think I'm a fairly patient person but I find the protracted wait for my nails to dry quite wearying. There have been countless occasions in salons and at home where, having sat around for ages, quite literally watching paint dry, I've put on my socks or attempted to rescue something from my pocket and seen the whole painstaking process rendered null and void by a smudge, dent or smear. It's why I often opt for gel nails, which are rock hard as soon as they're baked on with a UV lamp; one can get up and not spend the next few hours avoiding any situation that demands even basic dexterity, like some spoilt princess not wanting to get her hands dirty. And so while I often baulk at beauty press releases describing some reinvention of the wheel as 'life-changing', in its own small way, Seche Vite top coat has changed mine.

It's a clear polish, launched in 1991 primarily for salon use, that looks much like any other, and works in the same way: you simply apply over colour polish to shine and protect your manicure. But unlike the rest, Seche Vite dries in around a minute, and within five is usually hard enough to allow normal life to resume. It works infinitely better than those fast-drying sprays you can get, doesn't dry out in the bottle and weld the lid shut, and adds more gleaming shine than many traditional top coats. It's not perfect. I personally find that Seche Vite shortens the lifespan of my manicure by about a day (the polish tends to shrink back a fraction underneath it) and so if I'm enjoying a lazy evening, painting my nails in front of the telly with someone on hand to boil the kettle, then I'll use something else – perhaps a top coat by Revlon or Nails Inc. But for quick changes on photo shoots, last-minute paint jobs on the way out for some fun, morning chip repairs and the stemming of ladders in my tights, then Seche Vite is absolutely invaluable. Nothing else comes close.

Exactly when celebrity perfumes first hit the shelves is something of a moot point. Sophia Loren, whose Sophia appeared as far back as 1981, has a strong claim, while the first blockbuster celebrity scent was surely Elizabeth Taylor's White Diamonds in 1991. Yes, Cher fans, the Goddess of Pop did indeed launch Uninhibited in 1987, but it had been and gone quicker than you can believe in life after love.

In any event, the fragrance that started the second wave, the celebrity perfume gold rush, was without question Jennifer Lopez's Glow. The scent, released through Coty, was just one part of a lifestyle brand – J.Lo – that was also to include clothing, eyewear, swimwear and accessories. Glow was to be a combination of Lopez's favourite scents, in theory a hazardous way to construct a fragrance. I mean, I love the smells of bread, petrol and the interior of an old lady's handbag, but it's not a *mélange* I plan to dab about my person any time soon. Fortunately, J. Lo's own favourites, including fresh, clean notes of orange, grapefruit, iris, vanilla and jasmine, miraculously fell into a light, fruity, floral accord that proved staggeringly popular. Glow sold not just to hardcore Lopez fans but became firmly established among a demographic that wouldn't know 'Jenny from the Block' from Jenny Eclair.

The industry saw dollar signs, and Christina, Britney, Kylie, Sarah Jessica Parker, David Beckham et al. soon followed suit with fragrances of their own.

Glow itself, meanwhile, spawned a number of spin-offs, including Miami Glow in 2005 and LA Glow in 2010, a timeline that sounds remarkably like the history of the TV show *CSI*.

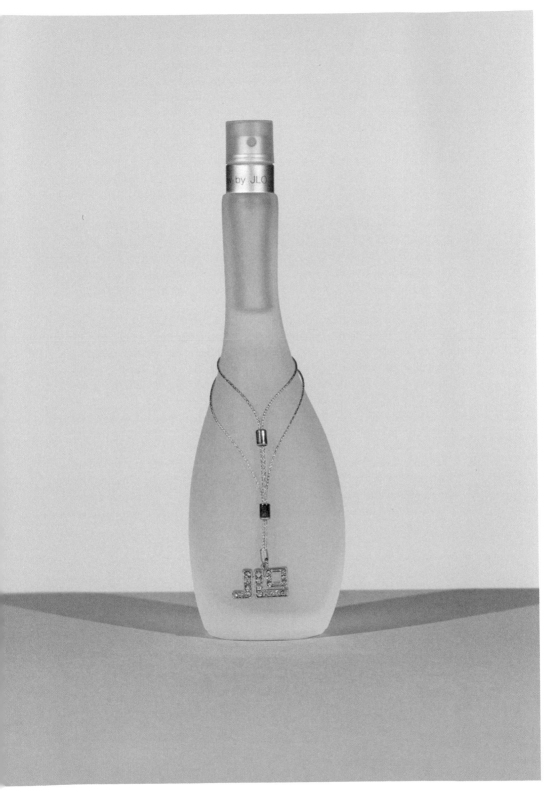

Go down to the bottom-right-hand corner of France, half an hour's drive north of Cannes, and you'll find the picturesque town of Grasse. It is the world's perfume capital, the very heart of the fragrance establishment.

Go down to the bottom-right-hand corner of London and you'll find the suburban vista of Bexleyheath, where Jo Malone grew up on a council estate, pretty much as non-establishment as you can get. Malone, who suffered from dyslexia, left school at 13 and followed in her mother's footsteps by working as a facialist. She would mix bath oils at home and began handing out a nutmeg and ginger concoction as a thank you to clients. It proved a shrewd career move. By 1994 she had her own shop in South Kensington and rapidly grew the business through the late nineties before selling out, first partially, then fully in 2006, to Estée Lauder.

What made Jo Malone such a refreshing addition to the industry wasn't just her background. She made perfumes a lifestyle accessory, a simple, usable everyday thing for people who didn't think they were into fragrance, who were put off by schmantzty, cloying scents. This was a new kind of perfumery, stripped down, utilising one or two notes where tradition demanded a complex tapestry.

The perfumes, or rather colognes, were literal: Red Roses smelled of red roses, 1999's Lime, Basil & Mandarin smelled of lime, basil – well, you get the idea. Admittedly ephemeral, Jo Malone scents are not a spray-and-forget deal, but need reapplication throughout the day. Uncomplicated, and like her matching candles ideal for gifting, the fragrances complement the wearer rather than announce or define them.

In 2011, the terms of her deal with Lauder having locked her out of the industry for five years, Malone returned with Jo Loves. In terms of structure, the scents this time are a little more ambitious than her originals, a little richer and more complex. What she has not bettered is the iconic Jo Malone packaging. Those smart cream boxes, tied in black grosgrain, are as much a part of the Jo Malone iconography as the scents themselves. Whether presented at a posh dinner party, on a wedding or Mother's Day, they are simply never, ever unwelcome.

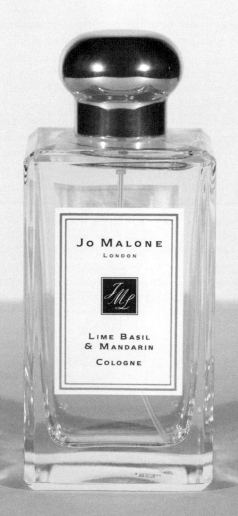

I have rarely wanted a product more than I did Eve Lom Cleanser. Launched quietly in 1985 for Czech facialist Lom to use on her celebrity and society clientele, this solid balm cleanser finally became a cult hit in 1993. And how. The sudden buzz around it was extraordinary for something packed in cheap white plastic, that cost an unprecedented amount of money for a mere make-up remover, and that, inside, smelled like a cross between boozy mince pies and antiseptic graze ointment. Eve Lom's cleanser was radically different from anything else on the market. No lather, no perfume, no need for cotton wool, this cleansing balm came with a muslin cloth and strict instructions for a convoluted massage technique that made you feel tired just reading the leaflet. The medicinal-seeming cleanser was to be massaged in meticulously to dissolve away make-up and dirt, then melted with repeated hot muslin compresses, before being wiped away. The ritual ended with a cold compress, like those used by old Hollywood starlets.

Despite its cost, this wasn't about luxury, it was about stripping back the fripperies and putting some serious graft into your skincare. But through word of mouth, rave reviews from beauty editors, as well as rumours it was loved by Nigella Lawson, Sophie Dahl and her supermodel colleagues, Dickins & Jones sold out fast, causing one of the only genuine beauty waiting lists in history (you can reliably ignore reports of others, they're almost invariably just a combination of PR spin, sensationalist journalism and outright cobblers). For me, Lom's philosophy was not a tough sell. I had already long since discovered for myself that the only way to cleanse and perform daily exfoliation was with a hot cloth. But Lom convinced a nation of beauty lovers in a way no one else had been able. With one little pot of solid, oily cleanser, she'd not only launched an empire, she'd begun a hot cloth cleansing revolution.

The Cleanser remains a bestseller in the Eve Lom range, acquired by Space NK several years ago. And I believe its continued success is deserved.

I would normally caution against using skincare containing mineral oil, especially if your skin is oily (mine is dry and therefore happy to drink anything you care to throw at it). But Eve Lom Cleanser appears to be an exception to the rule. I've seen remarkable results on oily, decongested, problem skin and rarely any adverse effects. Not that anyone need rush straight out to buy a cleanser costing the same as a decent wine and a good steak. Lom's legacy is more than just a product, and if you take nothing else from it, do start using a hot cloth (a muslin if sensitive, a flannel if not) to remove cleansing oil or balm cleanser of any reasonable quality. Your skin will display its gratitude within seven days, I promise.

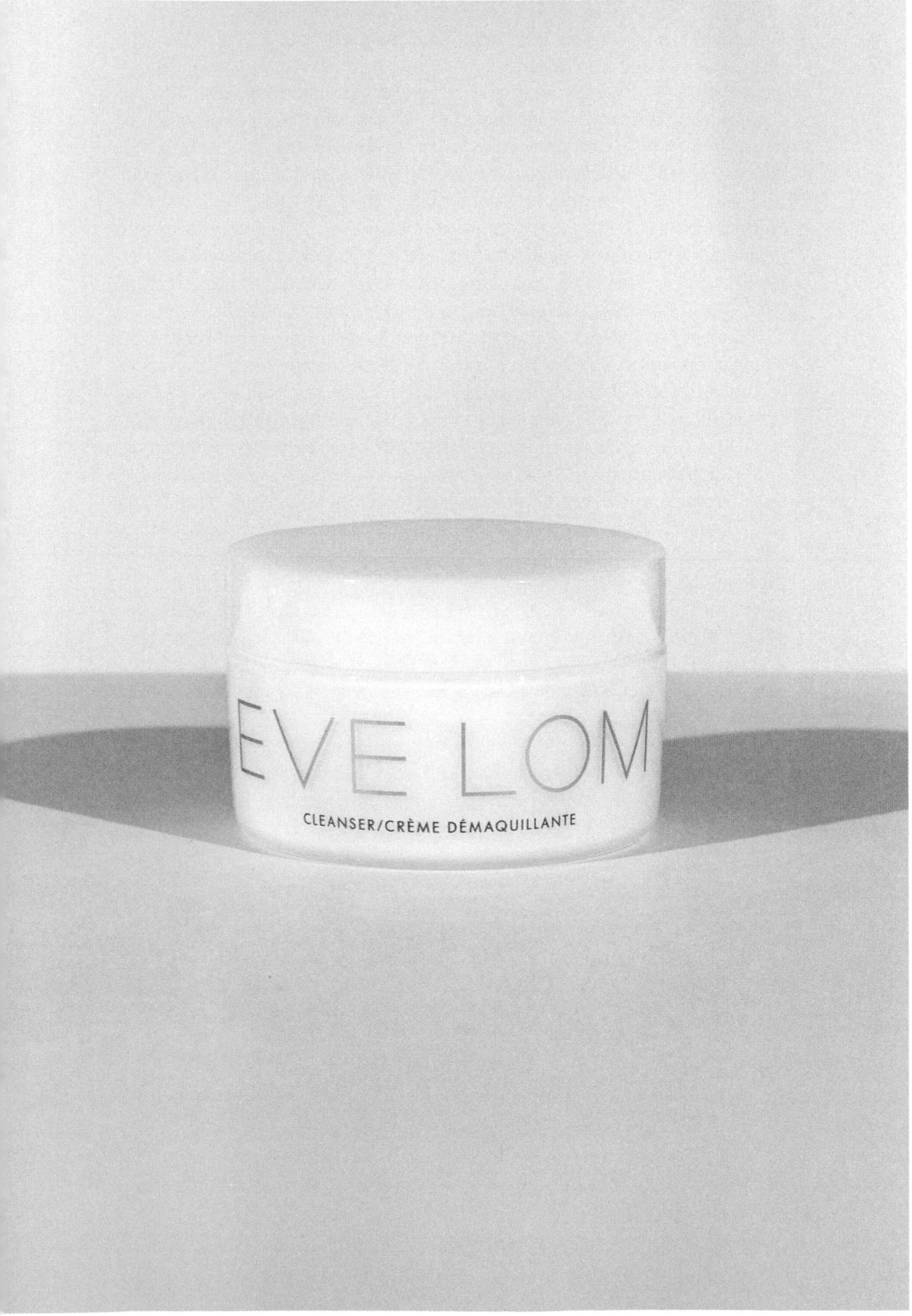
EVE LOM
CLEANSER/CRÈME DÉMAQUILLANTE

Perfume in a can might sound like a gimmick. In the case of Yves Saint Laurent's Rive Gauche, it was much more.

Launched two years after Apollo 11 and ten after the Pill, Rive Gauche showed up after a decade of increasing sexual freedom and the exploration of new frontiers. Its appearance reflected the growing commercial muscle of a generation of women striving to escape lingering, restrictive, pre-war gender roles and live an independent, modern and mobile life. To that point, perfumes had habitually been presented in decorative glass bottles, heavy or fragile, invariably designed to catch the eye of the wearer's husband – the provider – as much as the wearer herself, thereafter to live prettily on the dressing table from which the homemaking missus would rarely have cause to stray far.

But if Rive Gauche was to be a gift, it was one a woman would buy for herself. The vivid, cylindrical pop-deco canister, black and chrome bands on an azure ground, begged to have its top popped for a quick post-café-lunch dosing before being thrown back in a handbag for whatever adventure the afternoon might bring. The stripes also referenced the apparel of the hip poets, musicians and Gauloises-toting scenesters who languidly patrolled the Seine's Left Bank, the alternative, arty quarter from which the scent (and parent fashion label) took its name. That gorgeous little spray can may have hinted at disposability, but even after it's spritzed its last, this remains one container that belongs on the mantelpiece, never the bin.

However impressive the bottle, though, it couldn't and still can't steal the show from what lay inside. The wonderful scent is a floral aldehyde – arguably all-time best of its type (Chanel No 5 vs Rive Gauche is quite the fight) – meaning it has a cleanliness that's not wafty or ephemeral but unashamedly artificial and durable. I associate Rive Gauche, irrevocably, with a specific red satiny pair of my mother's knickers (yes, clean), impregnated indelibly with the stuff and scrunched up like a security blanket in my toddler hand as I waddled around the house, thumb in mouth, inhaling the scent, and maybe the very idea of sophisticated 1970s-style womanhood.

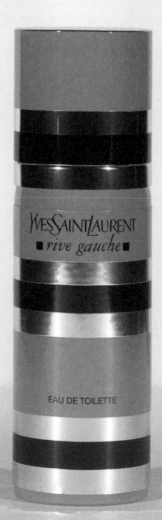

I'm a sucker for a skin brightening product, mostly because my complexion is prone to dullness but also because I find anything that adds light to skin of any tone is flattering and adds a pretty softness from which anyone over 25 can benefit. Brightening products are common these days, but when I first encountered Le Blanc at just 15 years old, it stood alone in a market crowded with flat, matte bases. It was so unlike anything else that I wouldn't have had the first idea how to use it, were it not for the fact that I got to watch legendary make-up artist Paul Starr apply it to model Eugenie Vincent on a fashion shoot for the late, great photographer Brad Branson. I sat on the stool next to him, trying to be invisible, as he brushed the white cream (as it was in those days – now it's a thick liquid) over her face, adding more at the cheekbones, dabbing a little down the centre of her nose, warming the whole thing with his huge hands until the product fused with the skin, casting a white gauze over it, before the real business of creating an extraordinarily skilled make-up design on top. Even though this was my first photo shoot and I knew nothing of professional lighting, I could see, as soon as Eugenie stood on set, how the huge studio lights sought out the Le Blanc, bouncing off it, drawing out features and bathing her entire face in bright, vibrant light.

I still love Le Blanc now, even though it is surrounded by hundreds of primers with a stronger light-reflecting ability. Ironically, that is why it remains unique. There's no floodlit glow here; it's not the ideal base if you're looking for even the tiniest bit of sparkle. Typically of Chanel, it remains refined and unshowy. What Le Blanc gives Caucasian or light Asian skin is an overall brightness. It tones down redness, it curtails shine, it can be mixed with a too-dark foundation to lift it by a shade, or added after everything else as a spot highlighter. Unlike the silicone-heavy primers of today (this, it has to be said, is more talc-y), Le Blanc can be worked quite vigorously into the skin without coming close to peeling off. It also comes in that peerless chic packaging, of course. Let's never pretend that doesn't help.

Sometimes an idea is so simple and glaringly obvious that you wonder why you didn't think of it and aren't now lying in a spun-gold hammock, lunching on barbecued unicorn. Custom Color Drops are vials of pure liquid pigment (in an impressive twenty-four shades across all ethnicities) that can be added to anything – silicone, water, oil, gel, serum, cream or lotion – to give your favourite product some skin-toned coverage. They effectively mean that all your day creams and sunblocks can now become tinted, your concealer or foundation can be upscaled to cover more on days when you feel particularly shabby, the colour of a poorly chosen foundation can be adjusted a fraction, and even your facial oil becomes a sheer skin-toned base if you fancy it. They admittedly take a little practice to master. The drops are extremely concentrated, and too big a dose looks chalky. But when you get the hang of it, the possibilities are endless.

Who doesn't know how to tie a ponytail? You just gather the hair in a bunch, hold it securely, place a band around it, twist, and go round again. Easy. The problem is that in the process, you invariably cede a little of the tightness in your grip and the hair loses tension as a result. So how do you keep the ponytail super-tight and sleek without growing a third hand? You use a Hair Bungee. The name, of course, comes from the bungee rope. But if the whole flinging yourself into a ravine business has passed you by, think of those cords with a hook at either end stretched over a car roof to secure luggage. The Hair Bungee, deeply loved by top session hairstylists, is essentially this in miniature. Once one end is hooked into the ponytail (do it on the underside so the hook doesn't show), the specialised elastic can be pulled up and around as many times as necessary, one-handed, and the other end then hooked in by the first. With the free hand keeping the ponytail in place throughout, the result is neat, tight and fixed.

Another issue with the standard bobble on a ponytail is the risk of snagging in the tiny metal clasp. Resort to a rubber band and the catching and tugging tends to be even worse – like a mini-flashback to having your hair pulled by the school bully. Blax's innovation was to fashion bands from a smooth polyurethane that would slip on and off easily and without snags, but with sufficient elasticity to stay in place in the interim. They're unassumingly thin, but stronger than they look, and their reusability justifies what might initially seem like an unwarranted price tag for what is ultimately a packet of tiny plastic loops. Available in a variety of tones, the most expensive over time might prove to be the clear – since they can be a bugger to spot when dropped on the ground.

Two brands, two products, as simple as they are invaluable.

A perfume that's not a perfume; that's there, then isn't, then is again; that can apparently be smelled by everyone except the person wearing it, with whom they will all fall helplessly in lust.

Escentric Molecule's attention-grabbing 2006 scent sounds like something halfway between a mad scientist's dinner party trick and the kind of magic potion shilled in the back pages of an offbeat 1970s magazine. Rumours swirled about Molecule 01's shape-shifting, attractant qualities: that it was a pheromone, that it acted like a pheromone, that it activated the body's natural pheromones. The truth, according to creator Geza Schoen, was simply that it's 'not possible not to like it', though the perfume's quasi-mystical rep does perhaps have some scientific basis.

First, is Molecule 01 a perfume at all? Well, yes and no. Meet Iso E Super, an aroma chemical that adds a woody quality to soaps, detergents, deodorants, air fresheners, even tobacco flavouring. It's also a common component of many perfumes, notably Calvin Klein's Eternity, Dior's Fahrenheit, Perles de Lalique and Terre d'Hermès. And Molecule 01? Well, Molecule 01 doesn't feature Iso E Super. It *is* Iso E Super. Apart from some diluting alcohol, there's nothing else in the bottle. The idea was that, unencumbered by traditional balancing ingredients, Molecule 01 would insinuate itself more subtly than a conventional perfume, the chemical staying close to the skin, the velvety cedar and sandalwood note dancing with the wearer's own chemistry, phasing in and out in response to changes in body temperature. Because of its responsiveness to the heat of the skin, Molecule 01 can seemingly vanish altogether, only later to reappear. The whole effect, then, is organic, primal even; a suggestion – unlike a conventional perfume, unshamedly 'worn' – that the fickle scent of Molecule 01 emanates from the wearer themselves.

Furtive as its single ingredient may be, Molecule 01 has remained a big seller. Layering with other fragrances may help you tether it down; I just like my fragrances to be a little more dependable, a lot less tricksy. But Molecule 01 was undoubtedly innovative, cheekily deconstructing conventional scent to challenge the very notion of what a perfume could or should be.

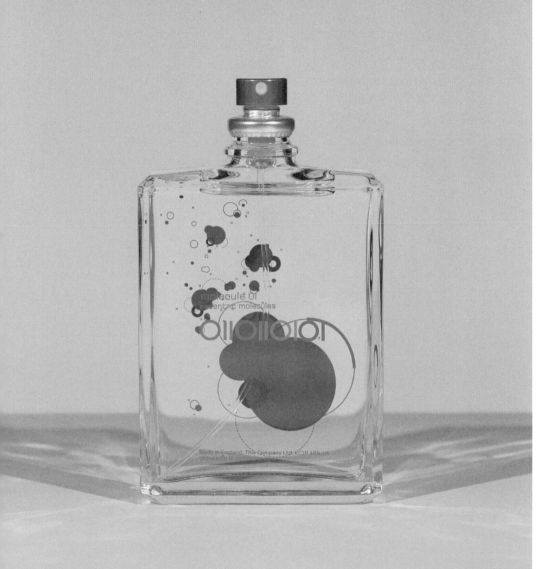

Top US make-up artist Jeanine Lobell's Stila changed the beauty game in so many ways that it was frankly hard to pick out a single product for inclusion. Her eyeshadows – packaged in thick recyclable cardboard and printed with a memorable quote from a great mind of the past – set out Lobell's stall on day one as a beauty company with a difference. Those clicky pens containing lip gloss, highlighter, eyeliner or concealer you now see in every high street chemist? Stila introduced them with its iconic Lip Glaze glosses worn by every nineties beauty fan and celebrity. Cushion packaging, so celebrated for its cutting-edge Korean technology and appropriated by Lancôme, YSL, Clinique and the rest? Lobell's Stila did it two decades ago with her Pivotal Skin spill-proof foundation for busy women on the go. Oh, and those girlie illustrations you see on the packaging of Too Faced, Benefit, Zoella, Anna Sui, Percy & Reed? Lobell and Stila did it first with their 'Stila girls', a collection of multiracial characters featured on an ever-changing roster of themed limited edition collections. I could go on.

But Lobell's legacy, I think, will be Convertible Color, a collection of universally flattering shades that not only brought back the unjustly old-hat concept of creme blushers, kickstarting a permanent revival, but reintroduced the notion of one product for both mouth and cheeks, allowing women to travel light and make up with minimal thought and effort (application is a breeze. Just dot onto the fattest part of your cheeks and blend). Lobell was extremely clever in her shade choices, too. The bright but extremely fresh, sheer and wearable colours – all named after flowers (Peony, a dusty nude-rose, is the most useful shade you'll ever own, while Poppy, a sheer red, is the most instantly cheering) – look good on every woman of any age or ethnic profile. Every make-up artist owned Convertible Color and with these pretty, streamlined compacts Lobell helped steer fashion away from the dramatic, sculpted cheeks of the 1980s, towards the dewy, casual-looking flush so many of us still find irresistible.

Estée Lauder acquired Stila from Lobell, then sold it on again in 2006, its heart seemingly not quite in it, the indie, quirky vision not quite translating to a huge multinational. I've rarely felt so sad about the loss of a brand, nor so thrilled to see it return five years later under new ownership, with the iconic Convertible Colors standing front and centre, wisely left the hell alone.

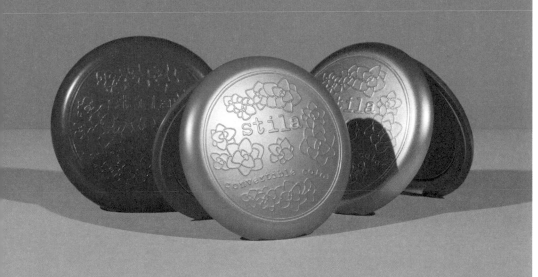

Yes, I know. It's actually Rouge Noir, just like a TV 'season' is really a series, and a 'bang' is 100 per cent a fringe. But in the case of Chanel's most iconic nail colour, the Americans for once got the better name. Rouge Noir, the European name, is literally accurate, of course. This black-red was developed following a request by Chanel designer Karl Lagerfeld for a red polish that would retain its drama in an upcoming campaign to be shot in black and white. Dominique Moncourtois, Chanel's director of make-up, didn't have a suitable shade in stock, and so he improvised, painting the model's nails with classic red, then drawing over them with black magic marker.

Inspired by his own gothic starlet creation, he put Rouge Noir into production to debut at the next Chanel catwalk show. Madonna rang the very next day and asked for a bottle, which she went on to model in her 'Take a Bow' video, a bullfighting melodrama in which her manicure plays an oddly visible role. In the same month, Quentin Tarantino's *Pulp Fiction* was released and its achingly cool heroine-on-heroin, Mrs Mia Wallace, played by Uma Thurman, wore Vamp polish throughout. What followed was something I've never seen before or since. Every woman wanted to own Rouge Noir, selling it out immediately. Magazines and newspapers reported the phenomenon, breakfast television featured items on the near stampede to obtain a bottle, friends had relatives scouring regional department stores in the hope one had been missed.

Even when the initial and unsustainable Vamp craze had finally worn off, it had already amassed such a devoted following that customers demanded its permanent return. After a fashionable absence, it was duly reintroduced, and settled into a position as iconic bestseller, where it remains. Its legacy on Chanel, and on the beauty industry as a whole, is huge. Vamp absolutely paved the way for other non-traditional nail colours, effectively broadening the spectrum of acceptable shades to just about anything. Without Vamp, we may well never have seen Hard Candy's ice-cream-coloured polishes, or Urban Decay's grimy metallics, or OPI's luxe jewel tones.

Meanwhile, thanks to the Vamp frenzy of '94, Chanel has become the only beauty brand to turn the tri-monthly release of a new nail colour into a global beauty community event. Black Satin (2006 – nails dipped in hot tar), Jade (2009 – medical scrubs green that made my hands appear wrapped in Prosciutto), Paradoxal (2010 – a glorious purple-grey that appeared to change colour with the slightest move of the hand), Mimosa (2011 – glittery egg yolk) and Particulière (again 2010 and my personal favourite, sophisticated mushroomy taupe) all caused beauty fans to temporarily lose their minds. Many have proved so successful they've been reintroduced into the permanent collection, while some exist only for extortionate sums on eBay. But none has yet come close to the success of this iconic nail colour. Or should that be color?

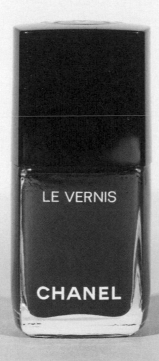

I've rarely seen a professional make-up artist's kit without a stack of Multiples, nor have I known a single beauty industry insider without at least one shade in her possession, and when I interview female celebrities and ask them to spill their beauty secrets, they so often cite these twist-up cheek and lip cremes as their go-to make-up item, that I'm almost tempted to ask them to change the record for variety. As a blush fanatic, I own multiple Multiples, naturally. This cornerstone of make-up artist François Nars's signature line is a wonderful, easy, clever, versatile, universally flattering stick of colour in every shade except naff. I use them on others a lot, particularly in their newer, matte format (I generally like shimmer-free cheek and lip colour. I daubed on plenty of shimmery peach Multiple in the early noughties but I also wore bootcut jeans and Playboy T-shirts, so I plead a temporary leave of my senses).

Unlike the fresh and pretty Stila Convertible Colors, Nars Multiples have a more polished, sophisticated look – in part due to a comparatively stiff consistency that allows more targeted application (though if you have the patience to do no more than smudge it en route to the pub, that works too). The colour remains so firmly at its station and thus requires so little touching up – once a day, max – that one generous Pritt-Stick-sized helping lasts an age. One caveat: as much as I've tried, I'm afraid I don't personally buy into Nars's claim that the Multiple is make-up for eyes, lips and cheeks. The sticks are, in my view, too dry and unyielding to be worn comfortably on the mouth and very few of the shades make for wearable eyeshadows for ordinary women. But no matter, because as a creme contour, blush, bronze and highlighter, the Multiple already does more than enough.

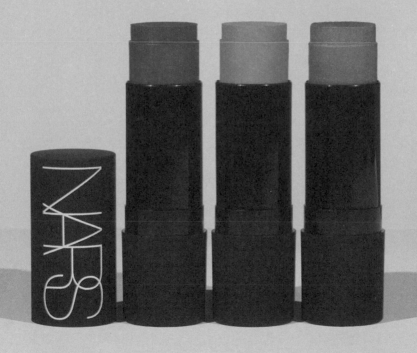

I still own my first black liquid eyeliner. I was 16 and it was a Dior, bought at unprecedented expense in Whiteleys (I doubt I ate much that week), for my first make-up job without my infinitely more skilled and experienced boss, Lynne Easton, to hold my hand and provide a comprehensive kit of great products. I've kept the liner in much the same way as someone might keep a baby shoe or university sweatshirt, because it reminds me of the beginning of a huge, if often rather terrifying and bleak, adventure that led me to where I am today. When I look at it now, I'm always struck by how much has changed in my life since I bought it, yet how little eyeliner has progressed in that intervening quarter of a century. Truly, innovations have been so few and far between that the ancient Dior looks much the same as a liquid eyeliner I might buy now in Selfridges or Boots.

The exception are these multi-award winners. Launched in 2001, these little pots of opaque gel-cream contain a rather crucial ingredient the dry, solid cake liners of the 1940s and 1950s did not: silicone. The inclusion of silicone – arguably the most revolutionary ingredient across all modern beauty categories – gave the liner just the right amount of slip to navigate the curves and corners of the eyeline with zero dragging, jumping or wobbling. The formula is, as the name promises, long-lasting, fade- and transfer-resistant (good news if you have hooded eyelids or hot flashes). The colours – and there have been dozens in the permanent and limited edition collections combined – are nice and solid. There's no insipid squid-ink black here (my pet hate in both clothes and make-up), just rich, sumptuous colour. And yet despite this, my favourite Long-Wear gels are actually the browns and the shimmers. They give the same smart definition as the classic black, only with an appealing, light-catching softness that flatters mature eyes. 16-year-old me would consider them a cop-out. 41-year-old me will take all the tricks you've got.

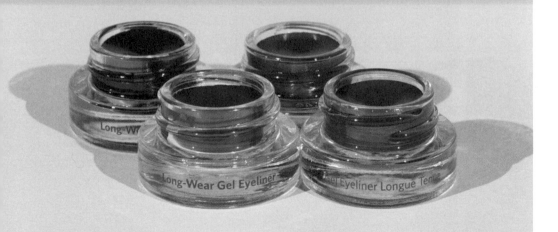

Kudos to whoever it was that named Creative Nail Design's revolutionary product after one of nature's most hardy and versatile substances. Rest assured, though, that unlike its namesake, Shellac's nail formula isn't based on the secretion of an exotic insect, just a blend of nail varnish and gel, with a mix of polymers and monomers that hardens to a high, durable shine.

When Shellac was launched in 2010, it exposed the weaknesses of conventional polish, acrylics and even gels. The process is similar for both gels and Shellac, in that the product is applied to the nail, then cured under a UV light. But Shellac leaves your own nail in better nick, as the process requires less roughing of the surface – beware the over-zealous manicurist, sanding you like an old front door – and in my experience the results are more impressive. Shellac nails emerge from the four-step process brilliantly hard and shiny, and, like gels, dry, so there's no need to get the manicurist to fish in your handbag for a credit card while you stand and waft.

Shellac's most important advance, though, was durability. CND modestly offers a nail that lasts at least a fortnight but my personal record is six weeks (major props to Maria at Daniel Hersheson). There's a certain pleasure in watching the little oval of colour gradually sail away from the cuticle as the nail continues to grow, unchipped and unpeeled.

As with a conventional gel, Shellac needs to be removed with patience and care. Nibbling, peeling, pulling and filing are strict no-nos: a patient acetone soak (CND offers its own oil-infused solution, and foil remover wraps) and scraping off with an orange stick is the only way to go.

Standard gels have retained a loyal following, some users reporting more durability and a shorter soak time than Shellac and I wouldn't doubt their testimony; much of an individual result is down to the condition of the nail pre-treatment and the particular talent of the manicurist. But if gels represented a big step in nail treatments, Shellac undoubtedly pushed the technology further and into the mainstream. Durably smooth and shiny, Shellac means women can put their hands through previously unthinkable trials and come out the other side still looking fabulous. As polishes go, it's totally nails.

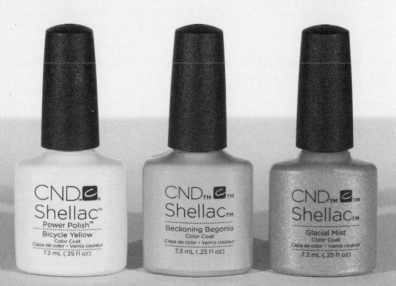

With Cleanse & Polish, Liz Earle did not invent the hot cloth cleanser. She didn't pioneer the use of plant oils to remove make-up, nor herbs to address skin complaints, nor the use of damp cotton muslin to remove dead skin. What, in my view, she did do brilliantly and importantly is switch on a generation of normal women (and by normal, I mean those who wouldn't set their alarm clock for 6 a.m. to get in an order for the new Verso serum) to proper, daily skincare rituals. Liz Earle's products make sense. They are simple, respectfully priced, they work for most people (I find about 5 per cent of Cleanse & Polish users experience a reaction or breakout), and Earle herself – having first created the range to soothe her own eczema – communicates their message with experience, empathy and warmth. She is, for many women I've met, the first recognisable face in the beauty industry, the person who convinced them they were welcome to join in, the only one they trust within it.

Which certainly isn't to say the product line is purely for novices. I am never without a bottle of Brightening Treatment, an almost instant glow giver that can be mixed into cleanser ad hoc. Her hand cream is the only one matte enough to stop me getting locked in the loo after washing my hands. And when I'm travelling and just need to grab one, compact bottle I know will get on with the job, I pack this, her world-famous, one-step, easy-as-a-game-of-snap, cleanser. Sadly, I don't share her love of muslins, and so they go straight under the sink, ready to use as dusters.

CLEANSE & POLISH™
HOT CLOTH CLEANSER

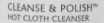

NATURALLY ACTIVE INGREDIENTS™
ROSEMARY, CHAMOMILE,
COCOA BUTTER AND
EUCALYPTUS ESSENTIAL OIL

Cleanses and gently exfoliates
for smoother, clearer skin

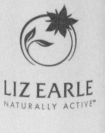

LIZ EARLE
NATURALLY ACTIVE™

100mL ℮ 3.3 Fl.Oz

Giorgio Armani is known for soft, smart tailoring, elegant evening wear ... and foundation. It has to be said that no one, least of all a beauty editor, expects fashion designer beauty brands to bring innovations in formula. Beautiful packaging, certainly; incredible shades you'd sell a kidney to have on your eyelids or toenails, yes. But state-of-the-art complexion make-up that smooths, brightens and feels like silk, not so much. And so when Armani (the beauty division of which is owned by L'Oréal) launched the fantastic Luminous Silk Foundation in 2002 and it went on to become the favourite of so many make-up artists and experts as to become cliché, the bar was permanently raised for his next.

Ten years later (eight of them spent in research and development), came Giorgio Armani Maestro, a genuinely new kind of foundation (or 'complexion perfector' as they'd have it known) that caused the entire make-up industry to stop and gawp. The racially inclusive Maestro was based on 'Fusion Technology', a blend of silicone and ultra-fine oil in which colour pigment is suspended. This gives tremendous slip to the whole formula and dispenses with the need for water and powder. In English, this means Maestro is exceptionally thin (it is dispensed from a dropper rather than a pump) and slippery to the touch, and light, non-chalky and natural-looking to the eye. Women – particularly those with oily skin – loved Maestro so much that within a couple of years of its huge launch, every luxury brand and its mother was on the fusion foundation bandwagon, flogging their own take on the original.

Personally, my Maestro use is confined to the faces of others. I simply cannot get on with a fusion foundation myself, hard though I've tried. I find the alcohol content too drying, the coverage insufficient for my preference (if I want a light coverage, I'd sooner wear a tinted moisturiser like Nars Pure Radiant Tinted Moisturizer or a balm, like Givenchy's phenomenal Teint Couture, than a foundation), the use of silicones too heavy-handed for my taste. And while there is no question that it was Maestro that changed the course of the make-up industry, I'm afraid I'm just another one of those clichés who really loves Luminous Silk.

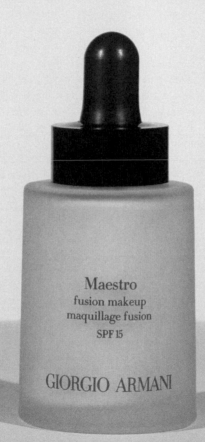

Few fragrances make perfume history; fewer still make legal history. But French designer Thierry Mugler's Angel did both, the second a direct consequence of the first.

Mugler's debut scent burst onto the perfume scene in 1992, like a drag queen kicking open the dressing room door after a bad show. Big flavours of fruit, candy floss and fudgy chocolate, tethered to a ballast of woody patchouli, created a new category: the gourmand fragrance – a scent that takes its key cues not from the floral, but the edible. Angel was inspired by Mugler's childhood memories of the fairground, though to some it might more strongly evoke a food fight at a kids' party. If a work colleague wore Angel, it would arrive in the office about ten seconds before they did, and for everyone who loved the puddingy fug, there'd be someone else discreetly seeking a cubicle on the other side of the sales floor. Nonetheless, Angel was unquestionably a complex, energetic and thrillingly constructed scent.

Among the admirers was venerable French perfume house Molinard, who refashioned its own Nirmala fragrance in Angel's image. The impersonation was too accurate for the liking of Mugler, who sued Molinard for plagiarism. The landmark court case was the first to claim one perfume had directly copied another and the judgement, in Mugler's favour, stated that contrary to the defence's claims, a perfume could be considered a work of aesthetic composition, rather than just the product of scientific process. Angel's claim was strengthened by it having demonstrably introduced an original idea to the fragrance landscape – that sugary, caramel note. Angel had actually been formulated at Mugler's behest by a flavour and fragrance company called Quest, that was not involved in the case. As it, not Mugler, was technically the only legitimate claimant, Molinard was not ultimately held liable for copyright infringement. I don't want to take sides, but since Molinard has remained a family-run business since 1849 and has been in the same premises since 1900, with a distillery structure designed by Gustave Eiffel, I can't feel too sad that a bit of copycatting didn't prove its undoing.

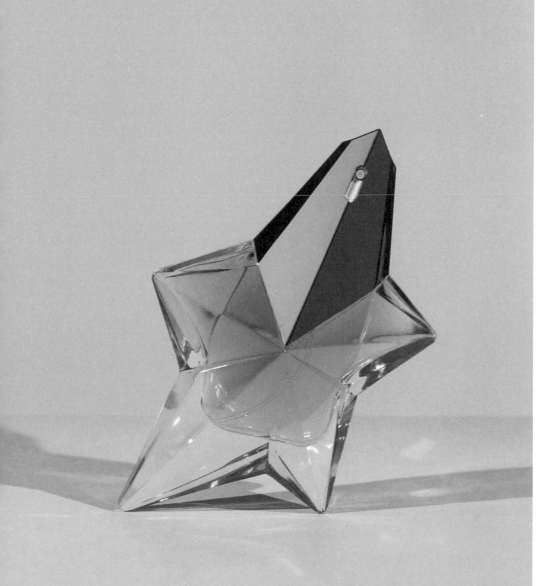

Perhaps surprisingly, given that I adore a face full of make-up, I find the current craze for contouring a bit saddening. It appears that not only were our boobs too small and our thighs too wide, now our heads are the wrong shape too, and need twenty-five minutes of our sleep time in order to be faceted like an emerald before work. And yet contouring is, quite simply, the biggest beauty trend I've known in my lifetime, particularly among young women (I think it was in 2014, when I watched a Japanese girl meticulously contour the back of her neck that I realised I'd finally found my make-up limit). I've barely done an event in the past three years in which a girl hasn't raised her hand and asked how she can thin her nose, or shave width from her jaw, and I confess that this is the product I'll invariably grab for the demo. It is, generally speaking, the contouring and strobing weapon of choice for most fashion make-up artists, and was certainly among the first to take the specialist contouring kits of stage make-up suppliers and adapt them for the mainstream.

Like any good contouring compact, it works on the basic principle that dark, matte cream creates the illusion of shadow, to slim and narrow anything prominent, and very pale highlighter – either matte or iridescent – pushes features to the fore, thus exaggerating bone structure and adding glow. As with any other, one paints the colours here in stripes onto facial contours, then blends exhaustively with a close-bristled brush or egg-shaped sponge to create the illusion of perfectly even features. But the superiority of Tom Ford's compact (apart from the characteristically glorious packaging) is in the colour choices. There are two colourways – one for white and olive skin, another for brown – and in each, the contouring cream is sparkle-free, taupe-tinged and without any whisper of orange (shadows are never orange, so avoid like the plague in the hollows of your cheeks). The white shade is wonderful: glitter-, shimmer- and sparkle-free, but high in shine so it attracts real light as you move. It's so lovely that I often end up ignoring the contour cream and using it alone. As do several top make-up artists, who I increasingly find are bored to death of contouring, and desperately praying it'll blow over.

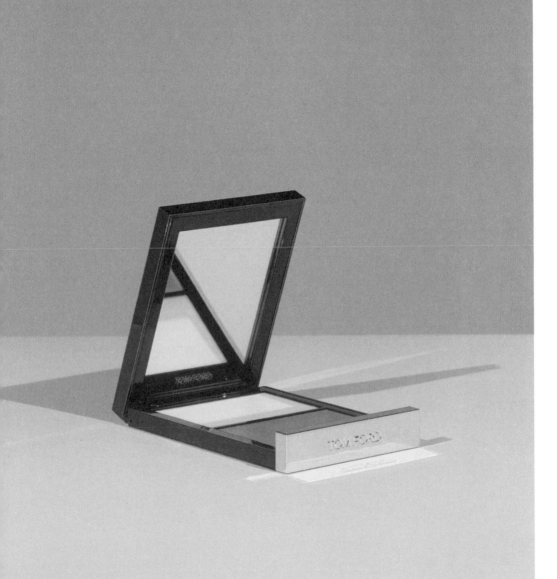

At the start of the millennium, there was a huge shift towards gradual, daily tanning products. Now, instead of going through the rigmarole of sitting on an old towel in your worst pants, carefully applying fake tan, you could just get out of the shower and slap on a body lotion and face moisturiser containing a much smaller concentration of active tanning ingredient DHA. This fast, daily top-up meant the tan neither faded nor looked too obvious and everything was literally golden. Except what if you couldn't find a tanning day cream you loved as much as your usual moisturiser? What if the gradual tanning lotions were nowhere near as rich and greasy as your gecko-like body demanded? (Asking for a friend here, obviously.) What if you were darker skinned than Dove, Olay, St Tropez and the rest imagined and you needed a slightly higher concentration of tan?

In 2014 Clarins finally proffered a solution. Their new booster drops could be sprinkled into any day cream (the Face formula) or body lotion (the Body formula) to instantly convert it to a self-tanner. A couple of drops equated to the post-shower gradual tanners we might use in winter, while three to five gave a more classic self-tan colour. Now you could continue using the products you really loved and still turn the colour of fudge.

In 1983, 21-year-old make-up artist Kevyn Aucoin was hired by Revlon – a brand widely seen, at that time, to be in decline – to consult on its high-end Ultima II cosmetics line. A year later he would launch The Nakeds and not only help reverse Revlon's fortunes, but change the face of the beauty industry entirely.

The Nakeds appeared in a make-up landscape dominated by unnatural and pastel shades that had nothing to do with actual skin tones – blues, hot pinks, greens, plums. For his reboot, Aucoin dispensed with all of them, and introduced what was then a revolutionary neutral, pared-down palette based on tones already present in the skin – brown, beige, taupe, fawn, ivory, peach and so on. For the first time, a major cosmetics company had launched a range that not only sought to promote a woman's natural look, but was suitable for skins of all ethnicities and undertones – something Aucoin had insisted on. The Nakeds worked with the face, not against it.

Aucoin's brainchild was hugely popular with fellow make-up artists (and consequently, A-list celebrities and later, the supermodels), who, like its creator, used the nuanced, subtle tones to make lips appear fuller, cheekbones more defined, eyes larger – in many regards, these techniques were the beginning of modern contouring that we see everywhere today. But even back then, The Nakeds look unarguably influenced popular taste, and by the time Revlon folded the entire Ultima II line (taking Aucoin's now popular neutrals aesthetic over to the mother brand), it had already feathered the nest for the likes of Bobbi Brown, Laura Mercier, MAC, Aucoin's own eponymous line and Urban Decay's own latterly influential Naked palettes. In some regards, Ultima II: The Nakeds was a victim of its own success: soon, everyone was in the neutrals business and it was no longer unique. There was something bittersweet about the fact that soon after arriving in London, I bought up a great deal of The Nakeds product line for next to nothing in the South Molton Street discount chemist, where it was dumped en masse in wicker baskets, while the brands it inspired were riding high up the road in Selfridges' luxury beauty hall.

The irony of all this, though, is that while the ethos of Ultima II: The Nakeds was to reveal a woman's natural beauty instead of covering it up, Aucoin himself was anything but sparing in the application of make-up. His 'natural look' was, in fact, a brilliant artifice. His was the kind of make-up, albeit meticulously and masterfully applied, that straight men who claim to hate make-up invariably cite as 'none', despite the fact that it took you the best part of an hour to pile on fourteen different products.

'What if the rest of you were as ugly as your nails?' Early advertising for Sally Hansen's perfectly named nail strengthening solution didn't seek to flatter. Launched in 1958, the treatment offered to fix unsightly talons, helping chipped, broken, splitting and bitten nails. Devised by Hansen and her chemist husband, Hard As Nails has been spectacularly successful ever since, selling around a million bottles a year. When giving my nails a rest between gels, I've tried many much pricier alternatives, featuring everything from plant oils to diamond dust, but really haven't found anything better than Hard As Nails. It dries fast and leaves nails feeling smooth and shielded. To moisturise the cuticle, I use it in conjunction with whatever facial oil I've got on the go.

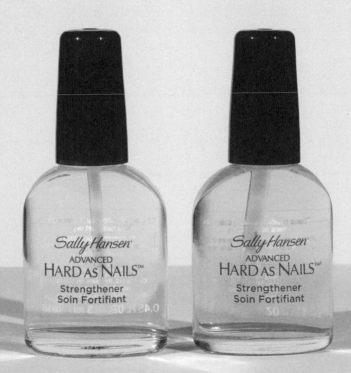

There was a time in the mid-1990s when it was my job to fold jumpers and khakis at Gap Regent Street, London. I was earning money to compensate for unpaid magazine experience and was so ridiculously broke that I'd frequently walk the two and a quarter hours to the West End from my flat in a dodgy street of kerb crawlers, and when I got there, could rarely afford lunch. Before this turns into some terrible 'woe is me' misery memoir, I must say that instead of eating on my break, I'd go to Liberty beauty hall and enjoy a thoroughly nice hour of not buying anything.

Then, as now, Liberty was full of intriguing brands you couldn't get anywhere else and along with the first Space NK in Covent Garden, was, I realise now, where the cult beauty revolution began. The newly landed Kiehl's and Nars had intimidating, downtown New York-type counters in the far end of the department, while much of the rest was lined with small racks of colourful treats. There was Philosophy with its cheek stains and Hope in a Jar moisturiser, displays of Stila Lip Glaze pens lined up like back-to-school stationery, baskets of fruity-flavoured lip balms from Australian brand Bloom Beauty, rows of Hard Candy nail polishes in colours only previously seen on paint charts.

And then there was Aveda. I had never before seen anything like it. Shampoo and haircare had always been divided into the cheap (Silvikrin and people like me) and the posh (Kerastase and rich ladies in Mayfair), but this was something else. Unlike the highly chemical hair products I was used to, these adopted the same principles as my favourite skincare, using plant and flower oils and essences to treat, nourish, even tint, the hair. The Aveda product I wanted most was Shampure, a daily shampoo for all hair types and even sensitive scalps, launched in 1989. Its smell was absolutely glorious – fresh, herbal and yet wholly unfamiliar – and was so unique that I began to identify it over the fug of fine, powdery perfumes as soon as I entered the store. Nonetheless, I'd never leave to go back to work without unscrewing the Shampure cap and inhaling it neat. When I finally started earning some decent money, it was the first treat I bought for myself.

Some two decades later, Shampure is an entire category in itself: it has a conditioner, (an excellent) dry shampoo, lotion, handwash, even a perfume oil, all capitalising on the addictive aroma of the original. And as much as I still adore it more than almost any other smell in beauty, it will always remind me of feeling quite hungry, of my stomach rumbling, and of wishing I had enough cash for a pasty.

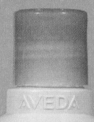

shampure™

SHAMPOO

SHAMPOOING

*above and beyond shampoo
with morikue™ protein*

*au-dessus et au-delà du shampooing
à la protéine morikue™*

8.5 fl oz/oz liq/250 ml ℮

I doubt many of St Tropez's legions of faithful slatherers think or care a great deal about to whom they owe their tan. For those who do, the answer is Nottingham's Judy Naake.

Naake, working as a beauty product distributor in the mid-nineties, was offered the UK rights to a tanning treatment then gaining popularity in the US. Because of its seasonal nature and the fact she already distributed fake tan products, Naake initially declined, but on subsequently trying a sample, she realised that St Tropez was a different proposition altogether and became an instant convert.

St Tropez, the first salon-quality tanning system available for home use, brought self-bronzing out of 1970s Coppertone hell by providing an even, convincing and more naturally fading tan. It could be applied without streaking and didn't leave the user with the palms of a serial Oompa Loompa strangler. The cream was tinted, which meant you could actually see where you were putting it, a big advantage over its clear predecessors.

St Tropez soon attracted the attention of celebrity customers, one of whom, then newly-WAG Victoria Beckham, obliged Naake to sign a confidentiality agreement stating that the entrepreneur couldn't use Beckham's patronage of the product for publicity purposes. Following a consultation, Posh left Naake's office clutching a bag of St Tropez. Fortunately for Naake, it was a clear plastic bag, the secret was soon out and St Tropez went stratospheric. Fake tanning is now a huge industry, with very many brands riding on the coat tails of St Tropez's groundbreaking success. 'Going for a spray tan' with St Tropez or otherwise is, mercifully, the new going for a sunbed (I long for these hideous things to be banned) and in the UK the use of self-tanning products to achieve an artificial tan no longer carries any shame whatsoever.

The excitement, however, was and remains at one remove for me. Fake tan's active ingredient, DHA – which reacts with the amino acids in dead skin cells to produce tan-like pigments (and smells like wet digestive biscuits) – does precisely zilch when applied to my resolutely pale skin. I've only once attempted a St Tropez treatment. It was prior to my wedding and suffice to say, I walked down the aisle with no additional colour but an odd yellow tinge where my bra straps normally rest. It turns out I am seemingly immune to all self-tan: I rub it on, it disappears. And since actual sun-worshipping is not my personal idea of either a fun or healthy time, it looks like I won't be turning tawny any time soon, by natural means or otherwise.

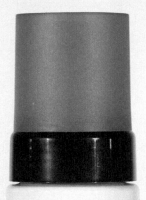

A handful of fragrances were so groundbreaking, or just so perfectly composed, that they still help define an entire category of perfumery. These are the reference perfumes, the scents to which perfumers return in the creation of new scents, to which pretenders may be compared for decades to come, and Guerlain is particularly good at them: Mitsouko remains a reference chypre nearly a century after its creation; Vetiver is the reference, well, vetiver; while at the head of the family of fragrances known as orientals sits another Guerlain masterpiece – 1925's Shalimar.

Perfumer Jacques Guerlain thought that vanilla had a powerful aphrodisiac effect, and on scoring a sample of a strong, creamy, uber-vanilla new synthetic, called ethylvanillin, he began to tinker. An apocryphal version of events says that Jacques tipped the new ingredient into a bottle of Jicky – Guerlain's even older blockbuster scent from 1889 – and Shalimar was born. It's a nice story, but a bit of a stretch; Jicky already contained a synthetic vanilla, and the sole addition of ethylvanillin would have created the perfume equivalent of sex with Mr Whippy. More credibly, Guerlain added citrus and resin notes coupled with deeper dusty, musky elements to counterpoint the vanilla, and Shalimar was the stunning result. 'If I had used so much vanilla,' reckoned Chanel No 5 creator Ernest Beaux, marvelling at his rival's balancing act, 'I would have made only a *crème anglaise*.'

Shalimar debuted at the Paris Exposition des Arts Décoratifs, a celebration of modernism in art and design (from which we get 'art deco'). Modern it certainly was, and shockingly carnal. According to Guerlain's grandson, Jean-Paul, the 'erotic' vanilla turned Shalimar into 'an evening gown with an outrageously plunging neckline'. Perhaps simply because it's been around for so long, some people nowadays see Shalimar as an old woman's perfume. If so, she's still a sexy old woman, and engagingly disreputable. As a saying from the twenties cautioned: 'There are three things no respectable woman should do: smoke, dance the tango, and wear Shalimar.'

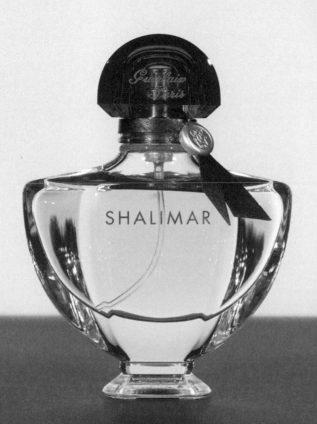

I love social media as much, if not substantially more, than the next person. But I also marvel at how quick the media is to credit it with the invention of beauty techniques that have been around since before most people held up a smartphone and pulled their first duckface. Over 500 years before, in the case of contouring, which was already being used in the 1500s to help theatre audiences read facial expressions from the cheap seats. Strobing, the 'hot new' craze in which women (and men) use highlighters and luminising creams to mimic the effects of light bouncing off young skin, is a technique that was used in the Hollywood studio system as early as the 1920s. Even its modern incarnation was born circa 1999, when make-up artist Val Garland revived strobing for the catwalk shows of Alexander McQueen (who had quite the soft spot for ghostly and space-age-looking skin).

The product development team at MAC, as ever, was inspired by catwalk beauty trends and developed a product for its new skincare range that would dispense with the need for make-up artists like Garland to mix white glitter or shimmer eyeshadow into ordinary face cream. Strobe Cream landed on my desk in 2000 as part of, it has to be said, a pretty mediocre skincare collection, and it shone brightly from day one. It's a very well put together antioxidant day cream containing tiny, shimmering, mineral particles to add glow and brightness to knackered or dull-looking skin. Tested on the hand, it can look a tad alarming, in a space-age sort of a way, but worn on the face it's an altogether more subtle affair.

The genius of Strobe, though, is its versatility. It can be mixed into almost any foundation or tinted moisturiser to transform it into a luminising one, or can be massaged all over as a glow-giving primer under your base. Dab over serious Saturday night make-up to add shiny light to cheek and brow bones, or slather on bare skin under a dash of concealer for casual Sundays in the pub. It is millennium beauty in a tube. Pleasingly, Strobe Cream remains cheaper than most of the very many products that have shamelessly ripped it off, and at time of writing, a new version for different skin undertones is on its way. I look forward to social media taking the credit.

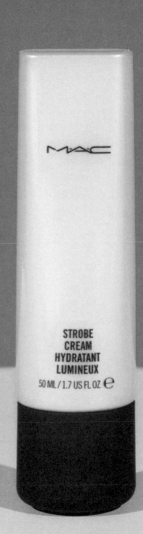

The evening of Tuesday, 27 March 2007 was a pretty big one for Protect & Perfect Serum. Until that day, it had quietly sat on the shelves of Boots, a modest part of the store's familiar own-brand skincare range. But then the BBC broadcast an episode of *Horizon*, which tested claims made in the advertising of various cosmetics. Under scientific scrutiny, many failed to live up to their billing, but one emerged with flying colours. No7 Protect & Perfect was clinically proven by scientists at Manchester University to repair sun-damaged skin and improve the appearance of fine wrinkles.

Boots website sold out of the serum on the same night, while, in store, shelves were picked clean in days. New stock disappeared as soon as it arrived and a year's worth sold out in two weeks. Before the programme, the company was making 10,000 bottles a month. Afterwards, it was turning out 24,000 a day.

But as well as brightening the skin of the nation's customers, the Protect & Perfect phenomenon had another effect. Previously, serums were at best a hazy concept for most British women. Most, if they'd heard of them at all, didn't really know what a serum was or what it did. But now, thanks to a glorious piece of PR Boots couldn't have paid for, a whole category of skincare had been thrust into the consciousness and – if they were quick enough – the hands of the British public.

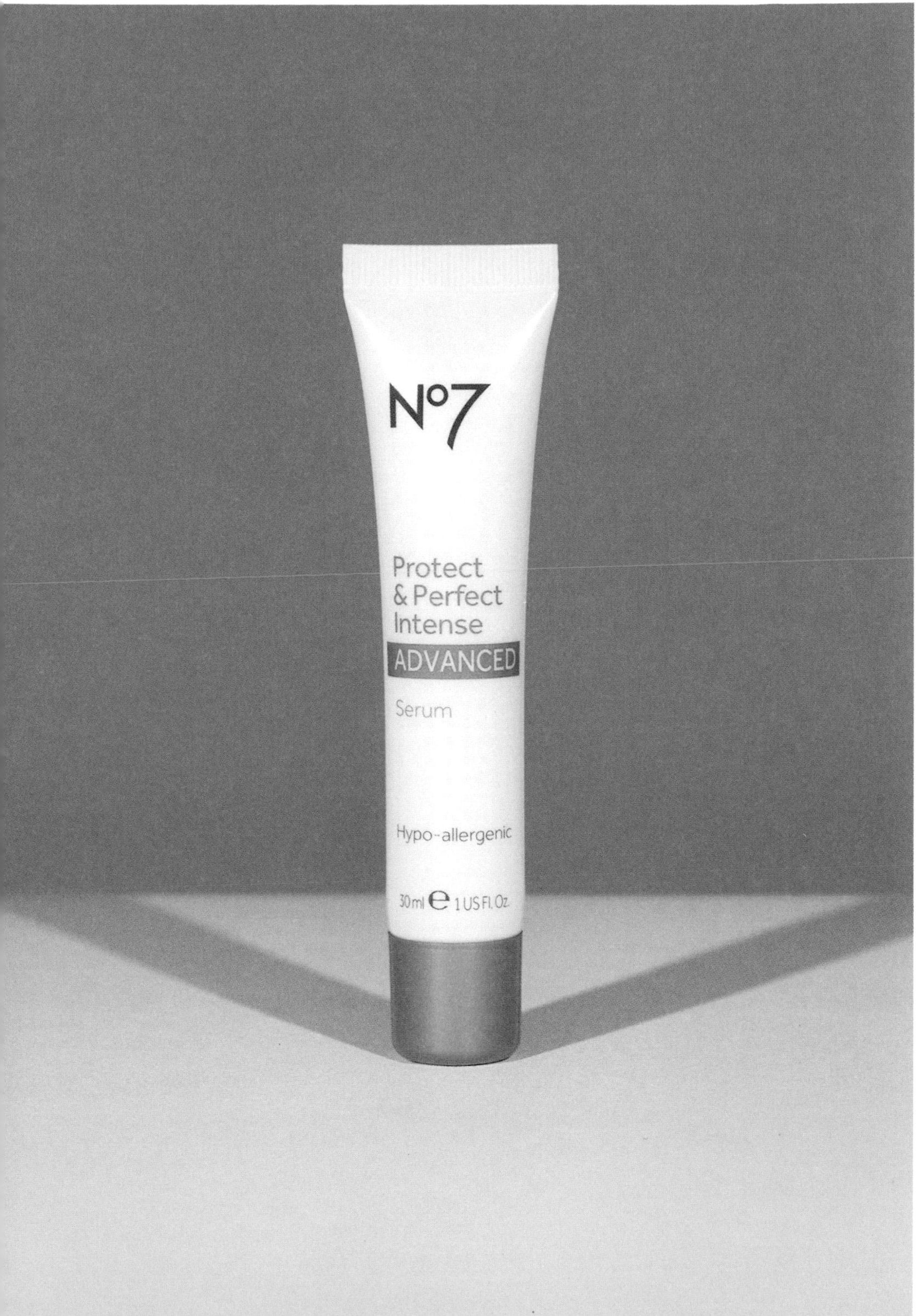
N°7
Protect
& Perfect
Intense
ADVANCED
Serum
Hypo-allergenic
30ml ℮ 1 US Fl. Oz.

The success story of Carmen Tal's massively popular hair product is really that of its most innovative ingredient: argan oil.

Argan oil is derived from the nut of the argan tree, endemic to Morocco. In a narrative seemingly de rigueur for any imported food or beauty craze, the oil has been used by local tribespeople for centuries – for everything from the relief of joint pain to drizzling on couscous. Chilean-born Tal discovered it during an emergency salon appointment in Tel Aviv, and was so impressed by its conditioning qualities she bought the company that imported it.

She began exporting to the USA (despite the name, the oil is still manufactured in Israel, it's just the argan oil that comes from Morocco) and argan oil soon slicked its way into the public consciousness. In 2007 just two new personal care products launched in the US listed argan oil as an ingredient. In 2011 there were 111.

From a user's standpoint, I must say, the Argocalypse has largely passed me by. Because personally I hate oil on my hair (unless I have nowhere special to go for the next three days and don't mind looking like a penguin in a Greenpeace appeal). It makes it really flat and lifeless. Friends, though, swear by Moroccanoil and tell me it makes thick, coarse and curly hair more manageable.

For the avoidance of confusion, Moroccanoil Pure Argan Oil is just that, and can be used on the hair, skin and nails. The product called Moroccanoil Treatment, in common with most hair-smoothing products (Frizz-Ease for example), contains silicone polymers, which are effective in taming unruly hair and adding shine, but relegate argan oil to a minor role in the recipe.

This is significant not just because it's handy to know what you're massaging into your scalp, but because it's indicative of how argan oil has seeped unstoppably into every corner of the beauty industry; barely a day goes by when I'm not sent a face cream, shampoo, conditioner, acne treatment, nail balm, bubble bath or mascara that proudly features the stuff. You can even find argan oil toothpaste. But in most cases the oil itself is present in such small quantities that its job seems more a marketing than practical one, so do read the small print.

I'm asked about primers more often than almost any other product. It seems that very many women don't really know what they are and why they'd ever need one, and I can't say I'm surprised. From the moment make-up artist Laura Mercier launched the modern concept of primers to the retail (as opposed to professional) market in 1996, and every beauty editor and celebrity make-up artist raved about these new wonder products, few actually stopped to explain why women really needed to incorporate yet another product and step into their already overstretched beauty routines. And so as someone who is primer-obsessed, allow me to explain why, for my part, I'd sooner surrender almost any other beauty product.

Primer is to foundation what undercoat is to wall paint. Usually silicone-based, it is there to provide the optimum surface for make-up application. You know those days when your make-up just doesn't go on properly and you have to wash it all off and start again? Primer prevents those. You know how foundation creeps off your face in the heat? Primer helps stop that. When the surface of your skin feels a bit uneven, bumpy and perforated because you've been a bit slack with its maintenance? Primer helps smooth it. To put it in layperson's terms, primer is the cosmetic equivalent of putting your face through a laminator, which is why I often wear it alone, i.e. with no foundation over the top, on casual weekends. It's generally colourless and therefore extremely easy to apply. Simply smooth (don't rub or massage) over moisturised skin, leave for a few seconds then apply foundation or tinted moisturiser for a much better finish.

Since Laura Mercier changed the game in 1996, virtually every brand sold in Superdrug to Selfridges has entered the primer business. There are primers for dull skin, spotty skin, uneven, oily, silicone-averse and dehydrated. The disparity in quality (seemingly regardless of cost) is quite extraordinary.

Some leave a horrible chalky finish on my face, others disintegrate into little balls when I apply my foundation, others are so thick with silicone that they just make my face feel weird. But this doesn't. It's silky, fine in texture, and doesn't leave skin so matte that it looks fed up. My personal preference is for its stablemate spin-off, Radiant Primer, but there's a version for everyone – mineral, hydrating, oil-free, sun-protective. But this, the classic formula, is where Mercier began her empire and effectively invented a category from scratch.

I have a deep and enduring love of nail art. While I personally have neither the patience nor the personality for striped, neon polka-dotted, decal-covered, jewel-encrusted, glittery leopardskin nails, I can spend hours gazing and marvelling at them on the wall of a nail shop, while my fingers and toes get their boring old Geleration or Shellac in block red or navy.

Nail art was born from Afro-Caribbean beauty salons, of course, and developed and proliferated organically, as technicians plundered their imaginations and perfected their art (and it really can be exactly that). Perhaps controversially, I feel that this, nail art's racial heritage, contributed to its particularly slow infiltration into the beauty mainstream which, let us never pretend otherwise, values young, thin, white females more highly than the billions of very different-looking women whose hard-earned money is just as good.

Gradually, from around 2010 onwards, we began to see nail art kits on Amazon, dotting tools in Topshop and decals (the tiny nail stickers to be trapped behind clear polish) in the aisles of Superdrug. Instagram tutorials and Pinterest boards showcased the millions of amazing nail art designs, and exceptional technicians such as Sophy Robson began to find themselves on the pages of *Vogue*. And so while Ciaté and its nail technician owner Charlotte Knight certainly didn't invent salon or even retail nail art, and nor would they claim to have, their ingenious and appealing DIY kits represent the moment when nail art went stratospheric in both sales and in status.

In 2012 Ciaté, having previously only manufactured polishes, launched Caviar Kit. The idea came from Knight, who, while on a magazine shoot, had created a 3-D design by coating the model's nails in adhesive and pouring over hundreds of tiny beads, as though they'd been dipped in cake sprinkles. She developed the technique for retail use, designed an at-home kit and sent it out to bloggers and press, who were quick to rave about it on social media. The kit sold out on day one, and went on to sell over half a million packs in its first year. Soon, Knight was designing kits for feathered nails, sequinned, floral, chalk-graffiti'd, shell-encrusted, glow-in-the-dark and velvet-covered nails and we, apparently, couldn't get enough. Other brands followed suit, but Ciaté's ingenuity and creativity continued to stand a long way out. Ciaté's kits (and nail polish advent calendar) are now an eagerly awaited feature of the Christmas beauty collections. And one day, I might even unpack a box and use one.

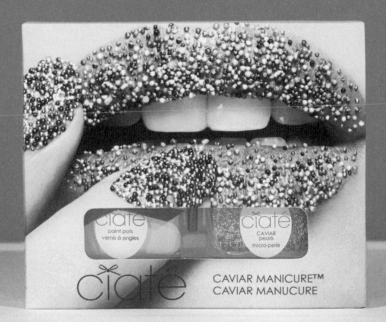

In beauty marketing, the appliance of science is everywhere. More ad time seems to be given over to lab-coated boffins (some genuine, some laughably not) introducing animations of magnified cells, pores, follicles and gumlines, than to shots of the products themselves. It's understandable. We want to know that what's going on our skin and in our hair is safe, justifies the price tag, and primarily, of course, works.

In the case of Allergan's anti-ageing serum Prevage, the science bit was its featured antioxidant, idebenone. Antioxidants fight free radicals, which over time have accumulated a charge sheet featuring everything from diabetes to cancer. That they also cause ageing, due to their oxidative effect on cells, is a theory that dates back to the 1950s.

Prevage was initially available only from dermatologists directly, though Allergan subsequently teamed up with Elizabeth Arden to produce a retail version, featuring just half the 'physician-strength' level of idebenone of the original. For the first time, a dermatologist-prescribed serum was available over the counter.

The problem is, though, that the free radical theory, while supported by most cosmetic dermatologists, has never been definitively proved. And so in turn it can't conclusively be said that the antioxidants in Prevage are actually fighting the right enemy. Moreover, Prevage's whole 'dermatologists only' shtick was a bit of sleight of hand. Idebenone is not restricted or regulated. Antioxidants are not prescription-only drugs. There was no reason, other than canny marketing, that Prevage couldn't have been sold direct to the public in the first place, and at the full strength of the original product.

But here's the thing: I wouldn't have included Prevage here on the strength of a sales strategy. I really love the serum's formulation, and take a praying agnostic approach to using antioxidants. The whole free radical thing might be baloney, but it might not. I'm happy to give it a go and hope it works. It's not all about the science.

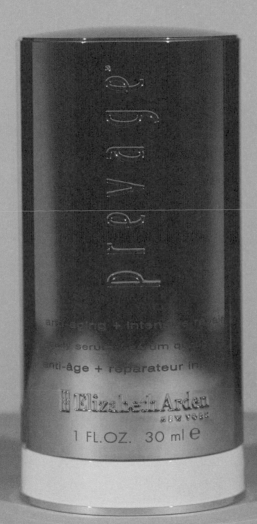

There are few expressions more likely to send my blood pressure into the danger zone than 'Real Woman'. This – usually applied exclusively to women with tiny waists, big bottoms, enormous boobs and, consequently, the kind of glorious curves possessed by *Mad Men*'s Christina Hendricks and no one you've encountered in real life, ever – is ostensibly an appreciation of more diverse beauty ideals (admirable and important) but in reality is just as prescriptive, unrealistic and patronising as wanting all women to look like Kate Moss. What tabloid newspapers, daytime TV shows and lazy politicians are effectively saying is that those implausibly proportioned one-in-a-million women are 'real'. Fat women, skinny women, pear-shaped women, women with a thicker middle section, women with neither boobs nor a thigh gap, women whose bums are flat and whose hips are parallel with their knees are not 'real', but mere imitations.

The problem with the beauty industry is not that skinny models aren't 'real', but that skinny models are all we're given. We are led to believe that physical beauty is the preserve of the young, very thin, usually white, able-bodied blonde or brunette woman when, in fact, it casts its net a whole lot wider. Women (and men) who don't fit the beauty industry's mould should know that they're beautiful too. A more diverse and inclusive definition of beauty needs to exist, especially, I might add, when brands are asking women of all colours, shapes, sizes and physical abilities to hand over their hard-earned cash.

This was the thinking behind the Dove Campaign for Real Beauty, which kicked off in 2004 with an exhibition and billboard advertisements in Canada, featuring ethnically, physically and generationally diverse non-professional models, and inviting the beholder to question their notion of female beauty. Public engagement was huge, and soon Dove rolled out the campaign across the brand and the world, featuring more gorgeous women, whose skin colours were as varied as their body shapes and proportions, and whose age range was broader than the industry's traditional 15–30. Since then, Dove's ongoing Campaign for Real Beauty has featured transgender women, strong and athletic women, women with disabilities and prosthetic limbs, extraordinarily smart YouTube videos on everything from deception in beauty photo retouching, to the huge disparity between how women think they look and how they actually appear to others.

Yes, Dove's priority here is to sell creams, soaps, shampoos and lotions. No, the campaign is not perfect. I wish Dove didn't share a parent company with SlimFast, and I do find it problematic that a few years ago Dove launched what is essentially a cellulite gel euphemistically described as 'firming for problem areas': it seems so at odds with what is an admirable and important initiative and a good-quality product range with realistic claims. But overwhelmingly, I feel Dove has contributed extremely positively to the beauty industry when it could quite easily have just continued to flog product the same way as everyone else. Whether you like it or not, advertising matters. Dove decided to do it differently.

And here's the thing. Even now, Dove is still the only mainstream beauty brand declaring such a diverse range of women to be worthy of the word 'beautiful', acknowledging that beauty exists in the real world, not only on the catwalk or red carpet. And so, in this one case, I accept the 'R' word with thanks.

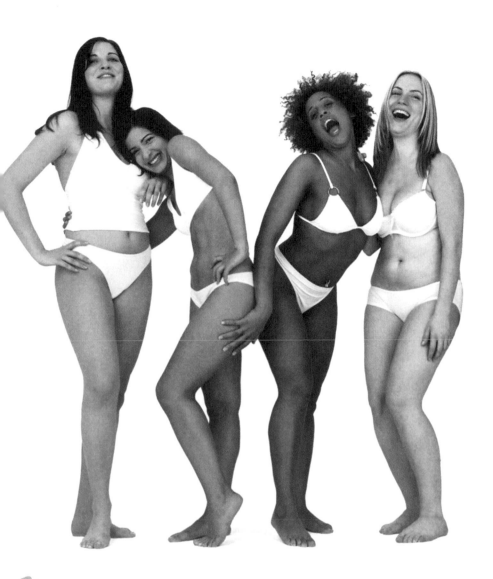

let's face it, firming the thighs
of a size 8 supermodel is no challenge.

There's not much point in testing a new firming lotion on size-eight
supermodel thighs, is there? That's why Dove's Firming range was tested on
ordinary women with real lives to live – and real, curvy thighs to firm.
After using Dove's nourishing and effective combination of moisturisers and
seaweed extracts, we asked if they'd go in front of the camera. What better
way to show the unretouched, unairbrushed results?

new Dove Firming Range

Hairdressing is in John Frieda's blood: his grandfather was a barber on Fleet Street and his father's client list boasted the moderately impressive likes of Ava Gardner and Eleanor Roosevelt. The third Frieda made his name in the seventies with the creation of the Purdey, the oft-copied mushroom bob sported by Joanna Lumley in *The Avengers*. His celebrity client list swelled, most notably with the addition of the still teenage Lady Diana, but by 1990 Frieda had tired of cutting and, having already enjoyed success with his own thickening lotion, devoted himself to developing a product line. No sooner had he put down the scissors than he was presenting his new brainchild, Frizz-Ease Serum, in New York. Lacking marketing dollars, Frieda was obliged to peddle his new product via public appearances and chat shows. It paid off, as the serum found its way into drugstores and two years later reached British shelves.

Despite a then hefty £5.99 price tag, Frizz-Ease was a sensation. By bringing the word 'frizz' into the minds of the public, the serum's name helped crystallise the very problem it offered to solve – taming hair driven out of control by humidity, heat-styling, excessive combing or chemical treatments. And by labelling it a serum and presenting the stuff in a dropper bottle, both unheard of amid shelves of mousses and sprays, Frizz-Ease presented itself as serious, scientific and unique.

Given that, in the face of industrial-strength attempts to get it to curl, my hair stays resolutely as straight as a builder's plumb line, the idea of me employing Frizz-Ease might seem as worthwhile as Jim Carrey popping out for a quick dental bleach. But such was the nineties vogue for flat, chopstick-straight hair that I embraced Frizz-Ease wholeheartedly.

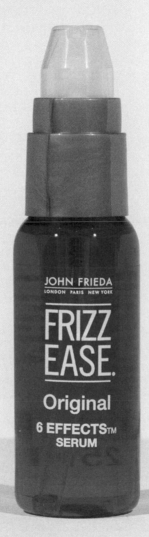

Confession: I have a thing for QVC, and always have. I can spend literally hours *In the Salon with* [resident beauty expert] *Alison*, not to mention waste countless lazy Sunday mornings on a wolf-print fleece I'll never wear and a state-of-the-art camcorder I don't need. But what non-QVC lovers may not realise is that Britain's leading shopping channel has a roster of genuinely brilliant beauty brands, and many of the cult favourites we now buy in Space NK, Selfridges and Cult Beauty actually got their big break there.

bareMinerals is one, and this is where I discovered it one rainy morning over a decade ago. Paraded somewhere between the Celtic Dreams cubic zirconia jewellery range and XXXL action slacks, bareMinerals caught my eye as a beauty brand that offered something unorthodox: cosmetics derived from finely ground minerals. I was far from the first, though, to be swayed by bareMinerals' shopping channel pitch. When Leslie Blodgett, CEO of then struggling Californian bath and body retailer Bare Escentuals, had first appeared on QVC in 1997, she sold $45,000 worth of stock in six minutes. Once the brand was firmly established on the channel, this would rise to $1.4 million an hour. bareMinerals was not the first to offer a minerals-based cosmetic range, but it certainly led the way in popularising a then niche concept and with it the idea that colour cosmetics could have health benefits – that they could add to, rather than subtract from, the natural condition of the skin.

At the heart of the bareMinerals range, and its success, was its foundation, a pot of dry powder to be buffed in tiny quantities into the skin. I personally find it a bit flat and dull-looking (their newer serum formulation is much nicer), but nonetheless it quickly found favour among those whose sensitive skin would invariably be irritated by conventional foundation, or who simply found it too heavy. bareMinerals' composition meant it was exceptionally light and caused no irritation. It was so pure, the company claimed, you could sleep in it. But please don't.

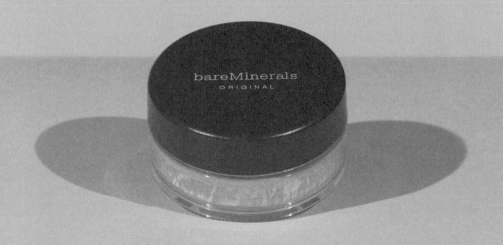

The story of the Clarisonic goes back to at least 1992, and a dentists' convention in Florida. Here the brilliant Sonicare toothbrush was launched, bringing a new wave of technology to the long-unchanged ceremony of cleaning your teeth. Eight years later the team behind the Sonicare (including engineer Ken Pilcher, whose CV also features avionics for the Space Shuttle) would sell their company to Philips and take the basic principle to their new venture, Clarisonic. It's not a huge leap – the Clarisonic is essentially a sonic toothbrush for the face and both claim to offer more thorough cleansing than manual methods (six times cleaner, manufacturers say). But it proved a staggeringly successful idea: by 2010 the company was selling $100 million worth of the things a year.

The Clarisonic provides a deep cleanse and is a great exfoliator. Though the company is careful to make no explicit claims about its ability to improve dermatological complaints like eczema or acne, it can, in my experience, be very good on oily problem skin. Some very experienced editors and bloggers in my peer group state they absolutely cannot live without their daily sonic cleanse, and their great skin backs up their theory. Others think the Clarisonic over-zealous and harsh, while a handful absolutely loathe it. I occasionally use the Clarisonic as an exfoliator and enjoy it, and I'd use it yet more if sonic brushes worked better with oils or balms, which are by far the best cleansers. But there simply isn't enough slip and friction unless you use a face wash, on which I'm resolutely unkeen. I believe that on dry or sensitive skin you're still better off with a terry flannel costing a quid.

But I do recognise that sonic brushes make people cleanse. The financial outlay, fun gimmickry, squeaky-clean sensation and ease of use seem to convert even the slackest of skincarers from their crappy wipes to proper twice-daily cleansing (and this, I suspect, is the true reason so many men and women declare the Clarisonic to be miraculous). There is real merit in that. And so while few products divide experts like the Clarisonic, I find myself languishing on the fence, leaning on the side of nuance. The advancing of age is a transformative thing indeed.

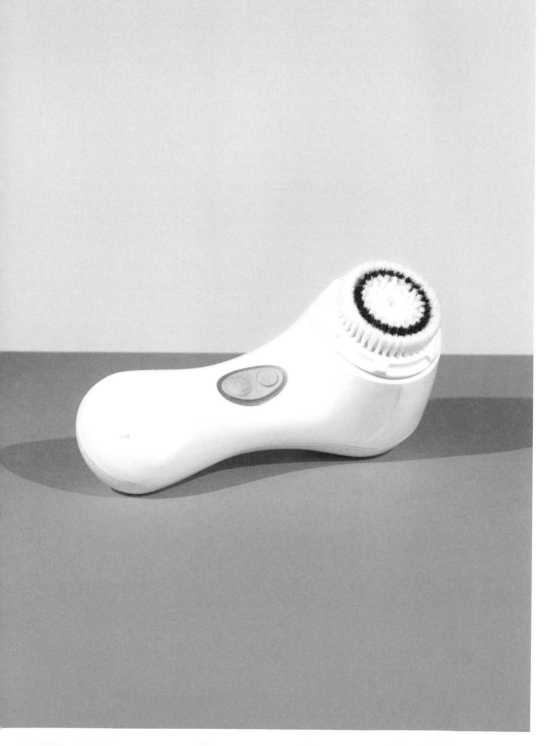

The early noughties. It was all about the Cat Deeley look – expensive highlights, St Tropez tan, beaded handkerchief tops, strappy sandals pretending to be from Gina and a Motorola flip phone. And it was an era of too-glossy lips that your poker-straight hair stuck to, thanks to the Lancôme Juicy Tube in the back pocket of your Seven jeans.

Juicy Tubes, a large collection of fruity-flavoured, high-shine lip glosses in handy, easy-to-apply slanted tubes that barely required a mirror, launched in 2000 and quickly became a status symbol, the thing the popular girls at school had by the half dozen. The tubes were translucent, showing off the colour within and screaming collectability to those who had outgrown novelty erasers and Beanie Babies. They also changed the fortunes of Lancôme. 'Till then a byword for mature French sophistication, the brand moved into the new millennium having dispensed with my heroine Isabella Rossellini as its face, and with Juicy Tubes made the Lancôme name relevant to a younger generation. Lancôme didn't only reinvent itself. Thanks to Juicy Tubes, lip gloss (a largely ignored product since the early 1980s) became the default lip make-up of choice, with every luxury and high street brand rushing to squeeze out a little of Lancôme's juice for themselves.

I owned three Juicy Tubes – Melon, Caramiele and Framboise – and while I was exceedingly pleased with them, I did feel like an impostor. One knows at 25 that one is cheese not chocolate, brunette not blonde, heel not flat, vodka not gin, Blur not Oasis, dog not cat and emphatically lipstick not gloss. And so while I'm glad not to have missed out on the Juicy revolution, my relationship with sheer, shiny lips proved fleeting. It's a testament to Lancôme's most legendary product that I even engaged in a flirt.

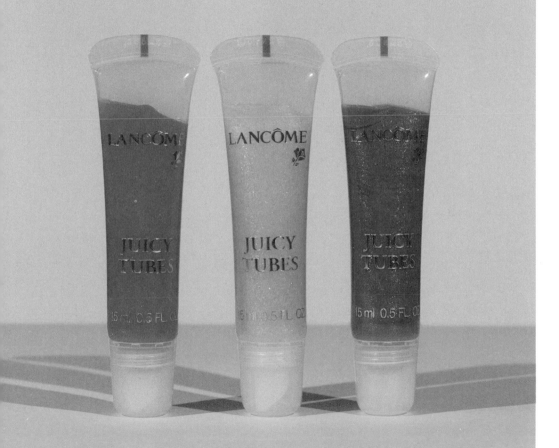

THE
RITES OF
PASSAGE

I have to say, Mr Matey was not a regular bath-time companion for my two brothers and me. My parents would have regarded a jolly, plastic, blue-goop-dispensing seaman as a childish and frivolous part of the routine. It's not that their approach to ablution was zealously puritanical – we didn't have to beat the dirt off with a birch stick or anything – but pimping the bathwater in our household was simply not seen as a priority, distraction provided instead by the kind of stupid, carpet-soaking, health-and-safety-disdaining games three tub-sharing siblings invariably devise.

But on rare sleepovers at a friend's house, bath time could be a more sedate and luxurious affair. Here I could commune with the obliging, rosy-cheeked sailor, seductively removing his jaunty cap before measuring the requisite amount of viscous liquid into it, then emptying carefully under the hot tap and replacing. Matey's work done, the poor guy would end up back on the shelf while I would lazily push the mountains of foam over the water's surface, watch the rainbow reflections and luxuriate, safe in the knowledge that the bubbles popping about me all came courtesy of the blue goop, and not of a brother's bottom.

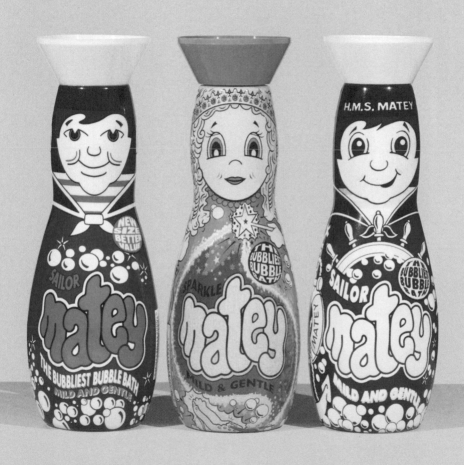

Oh, scrunchies. Those disgusting, fabric-covered hair elastics unfathomably trendy for five minutes, later seen on Sloane Rangers, market stalls, post-modern ironic hipsters and, frequently, on wet pavements, all grubby and still holding strands of their estranged owner's hair. Paisley sateen, flammable nylon, crinkled burgundy velour, buff suedette like a DFS sofa – the scrunchie comes in limitless guises, all of them abhorrent. But as much as I am loth to admit it, scrunchies really do have their use. If you'd like increased volume in your flat hair (and I speak very much for myself here), then just before bed, spray dry shampoo liberally into the roots but don't brush through. Scrape the front or all of your hair into a high ponytail resembling the stalk of a pineapple, and secure with a scrunchie. Sleep. Wake to increased volume, rejoice, and forgive the scrunchie its many heinous crimes against fashion. Then swear to confine it firmly behind closed doors.

Surely there is no guiltier pleasure than peeling off a pore strip except, perhaps, for the giddy and delirious watching of close-camera footage of blackhead squeezing on YouTube, but I know I'm an extreme case. When Bioré pore strips launched here in 1997, they sparked a huge craze. The irresistible idea was that instead of wasting precious cider drinking time on boring cleanse/tone/moisturise routines and seeing only gradual or slight improvement, one could simply stick relatively inexpensive pore strips onto nose and chin once a week, wait a few minutes, then whip off (much like a sticking plaster), taking every blackhead cleanly away with them. It was a hugely enticing prospect and, in complete fairness, Bioré pore strips did, and still do, almost exactly as promised. There was huge satisfaction in examining the used strip, hundreds of former blackheads standing to attention like a grease-coated lawn of grass.

The problem with pore strips, from my perspective, is that while it's gratifying in the short term to see plugs of solid sebum being excavated from pores, it is not all that helpful long-term. Pores are left open and exposed and will, at best, immediately fill up again and need re-stripping (no more than once a week please) and, at worst, be more susceptible to bacteria and infection. They can leave the nose area flaky and dry and are absolutely no substitute for caring for teenage skin with proper hot cloth cleansing, regular use of BHA toners, a non-occlusive (i.e. no paraffins and other skin-clogging oils) moisturiser and judicious removal of blackheads with clean fingers or extraction tool. And while Bioré strips are still affordable, the new incarnation of pore strip technology – peel-off black masks that work in the same way – are not. I've seen these sell for up to £60 as state-of-the-art Korean skincare innovation when, really, they are little more than Bioré pore strips with delusions of grandeur. If you crave the ephemeral high of blanket extraction, you're best keeping things cheap and unpretentious, and sticking with the original.

Banana Clips and Claw Clamps

My childhood 'look' was never complete without a side ponytail made even higher and bouncier with a yellow plastic seashell-shaped hair claw seen in *Girl* magazine and bought off the market. I wore it every single day, like a nan in a fascinator at a wedding. If playing dress-up, I might instead sweep all my hair into a banana clip – a huge, curved contraption that looked like something designed to immobilise bears. Both bananas and shells were everywhere for a good five years until Sarah Ferguson arrived with her terrible Sloaney oversized bows, and stole their thunder.

Nowadays, banana clips are practically obsolete and hair claws tend to be used for more functional than decorative purposes – by hairdressers to section while cutting, by women looking to hastily scrape back hair before a night-time cleanse and so on. One rarely sees anyone wearing them out, unless in the hipster zone of London, where 1980s revivalism is apparently without taste filter. I can understand more than many how hard they are to resist, though. I may no longer wear a banana or shell, but I still have a magpie-like appreciation for hair accessories. There's something so lovely about all the buttons, bows, ribbons, elastics, clips, crystals and colours that makes me want to buy them all and just gaze at them within the safety of my own home. Which is precisely why I should no longer be allowed near Fenwick on days 20–28 of my cycle, because I will invariably buy beautiful and extortionately expensive hair accessories that I will never wear because, well, I am no longer nine.

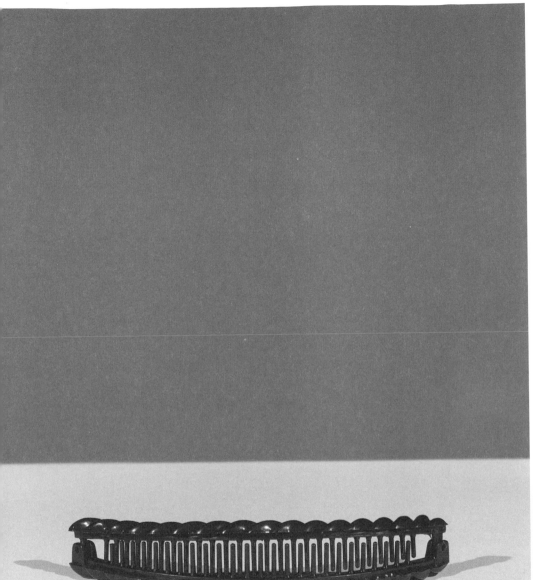

I think I love concealer more than any other product. Or rather, I rely on it most heavily; skin-coloured paste is not the most thrilling item, I'll admit. But I can't be without concealer because it's by far the most helpful and effective of all make-up, evening out skin tone, brightening under eyes, hiding spots, broken veins and discolouration. Literally everyone in the world – male, female, young, old – would think they looked better with concealer than without, even if they lack the inclination or skill to apply it. Like many women, Rimmel Hide the Blemish was my first concealer, and I must give it huge credit for that, if, at that time, for little else. As soon as we hit puberty and our pores began to secrete, every child in school seemed to dash off for a stick of this in its then standard salmony orange-pink. On my yellowy-white face, this weird shade (much like the colour of silly putty) made a feature of anything I was attempting to disguise and only propelled me to find something better.

The modern version of Hide the Blemish is far superior and comes in several shades, though not racially inclusive ones. I strongly recommend you bear in mind its name before veering away from spots and blemishes and attempting to use it on dark circles, where, despite what anyone might tell you, it is completely unsuitable (if you want a great bargain under-eye concealer, try Collection). Here, Hide the Blemish will blend poorly, cake over fine lines, make the area feel dry when it begs for moisture. This is a concealer to be plonked onto small, undesirably conspicuous blemishes, softened with only a few taps of your finger, then left to hold the fort, which it certainly does. And on the basis that it costs under a fiver, I think that's contribution enough.

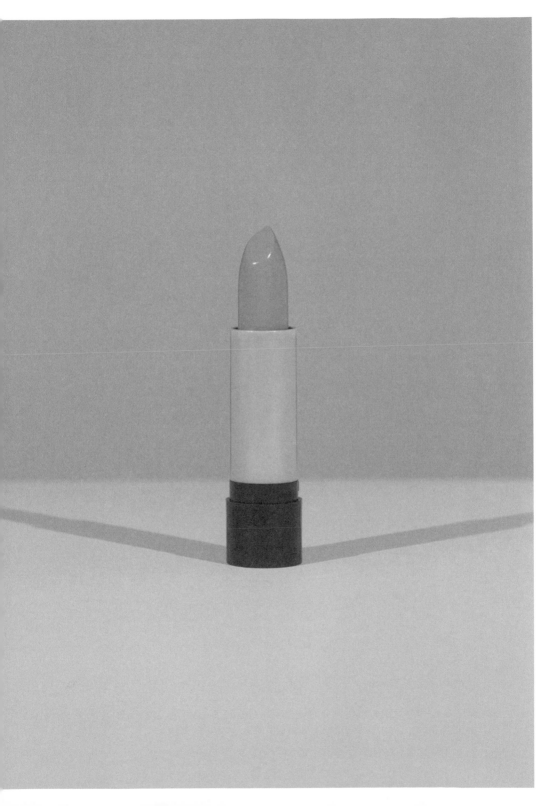

The problem with first foundations is that one always acquires them probably ten, but definitely at least five, years too early. This is because the teenage condition will not acknowledge that skin is the most evenly toned and healthy it will ever look in its life and insists on hiding it under a thick layer of poorly matched stucco. If I could step into my childhood now and extricate the 12-year-old me from my (espresso brown) bathroom one Monday morning before school, I would – if only to prevent me from discovering a glass bottle of Mary Quant foundation in my mother's make-up hamper. I slapped on the liquid with the plastic paddle applicator as though spreading meat paste on sliced white. No blending, no pausing to check the suitability of colour, no moisturising even.

And so off I went to school, so in love with the idea of wearing grown-up foundation that I saw nothing the matter with looking like surgical dressing. In fairness and in hindsight, there was nothing inherently worse in Mary Quant foundation than in any other foundation of the late 1980s (I think I went for Almay next, then Miss Selfridge; neither was an improvement), it just happened to be in the wrong hands at very much the wrong time. It was years before I discovered Clinique Superbalanced Foundation, in an identical bottle. The texture was better, the colour truer, and yet I still really had no business wearing it. Putting up barriers is part of the uniquely confusing period of adolescence. I wish we didn't so often make them physical.

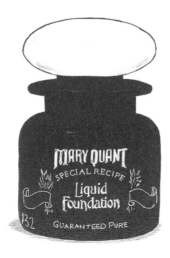

To be honest, brand is pretty unimportant here, but Country Born sprang first to mind from an array of generic 1980s manufacturers selling huge Swarfega-esque tubs of lurid-coloured hair gel for about 79p. As teens, we'd dip our glittery combs and brushes directly into the slimy, cauldron-like containers and rake them through our terrible mullet haircuts, creating stiff, distinct stripes that flaked onto our school cardigans as the day wore on. Girls with highly coveted spiral perms drenched their wet curls with the stuff, thus preventing them from ever drying and fluffing, like guillemots after an oil-spill disaster. A breaktime downpour caused the gel to run into your eyes and semi-glue them shut. I can still just about smell the chemical, sticky aroma now: it was the smell of school discos, of wet, clumsy snogs with fit boys during 'She's Like the Wind', of a hot, overcrowded coach trip to Rhineland. Delicious.

I believe strongly that no skincare regime is fully beneficial without regular exfoliation, and rely heavily on it for keeping my own skin looking its best. I use a wet flannel twice a day and have done for decades, an Alpha Hydroxy Acid liquid two to four times a week and perhaps the odd exfoliating mask during winter, when my skin can look a little grey. All are a million miles away from this, the star product from the UK's first ever exfoliant brand; my first ever exfoliant, and, I believe, the scrub that helped make the act of removing dead skin a mass-market phenomenon.

Aapri launched in 1985 with a granular cream made from coarse-ground apricot kernels in a creamy aloe, vitamin E and apricot kernel oil base, and sold for a mere one-pound-something in every high street chemist or supermarket. It was to be used as a face wash, the granules lifting off dirt, make-up and dead skin in readiness for face cream (serum didn't even exist then – certainly not for the hoi polloi), then rinsed off. Something about Aapri sparked the nation's imagination, and I doubt it was the naff-even-by-1980s-standards logo and packaging. Within a year, it felt as though everyone used Aapri and we were a nation of scrubbers. Clearly, the industry has developed the exfoliation market hugely since then. We now have everything, from crappy microbead face washes to sophisticated microdermabrasion kits previously only available in dermatologists' offices.

Aapri has been so off-radar in all this time that I must admit I assumed it had gone. It was only during the research for this book that I discovered it was still available via independent chemists. I bought some, tried it for the first time in decades and although I still believe granular scrubs are less thorough, even and kind than textured face cloths and acid toners (I've seen other granular scrubs under a microscope and believe me, it's not pretty), I will say that it's really not half bad. It still smells lovely and leaves skin softened and smoothed.

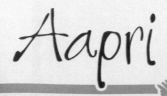

Aapri

EXFOLIATING FACIAL
scrub cream
formulated with natural apricot
exfoliants for healthy skin

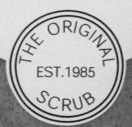

THE ORIGINAL

EST.1985

SCRUB

ideal for normal/oily skin
150 ml ℮ 5.0 fl.oz

It's hard to overstate the pervasiveness of perms in the seventies, eighties and early nineties. I barely exaggerate when I say that the permanent wave was the default hairstyle for any grown woman not going for a Lady Di. All hair salons stank to high heaven of perming solution (imagine, if you will, a particularly pungent dog fart, only wetter) and each must have had to keep a stock of 1,500 rollers to meet an average Saturday's demands. For schoolchildren – of any gender – one's first perm (some time between 11 and 14) represented a great stride into a life of maturity, sophistication, popularity and a guaranteed card on Valentine's Day. While my first perm – or as I look back on it, the worst hair I have ever seen with my eyes – was done in a salon (apparently an expensive professional was needed to achieve the look of hosed-down Tina Turner), many of my peers got theirs via a DIY box of Toni. This was a kit containing rollers, roller papers (much like Rizlas) and all the requisite chemicals, used by the more dexterous mums and mobile hairdressers of the day to achieve an affordable permanent wave. The enclosed leaflet explained how different roller sizes and formations could be harnessed to create distinctive looks, and yet whichever you requested, or however skilful your practitioner, you emerged from any Toni with something between a Kevin Keegan and a King Charles II.

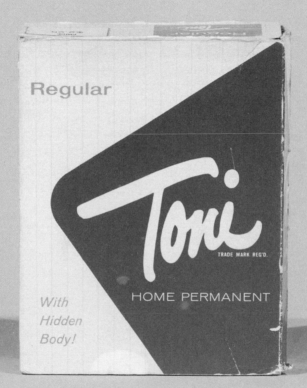

'Men can't help acting on Impulse' is one of the more memorable ad slogans of my childhood. And it made Impulse perfumed body spray a roaring success with young women, especially those in my school, who sprayed it with such abandon that the padded beams of the school gymnasium reeked permanently of synthetic pink flowers and musk. But in me, Impulse and its catchy slogan stirred something of a political awakening. While I certainly can't deny that I thought about boys almost constantly as a teenager, swotting in teen mags for pulling techniques, snogging the occasional mirror in preparation for the real thing, I somehow knew even then that Impulse's message of wearing beauty products to attract the attention of male suitors didn't really chime with my developing worldview. Nothing wrong with attempting to pull anyone, of course, but it did rather take the fun out of beauty which was and largely remains, for me, an almost entirely selfish pleasure.

Thirty years on, the same Impulse message remains a banker for the brand. Despite extensive modernisation of packaging, spokespeople, target audience and much improvement in fragrance (from the original line-up, only Hint of Musk remains), the notion of romance and 'capturing female allure' remain at the heart of Impulse's mission, and it continues to do the job exceptionally well. It is the UK and Ireland's bestselling body spray – bigger than all other body sprays put together, and all power to them. Personally, I can't quite understand the purpose or appeal of any body spray, regardless of brand values. My preference is always for a fairly neutral unisex antiperspirant like Dove or Vaseline Intensive Care, layered under a generous spritz of perfume. And my partner is mustard keen, all the same.

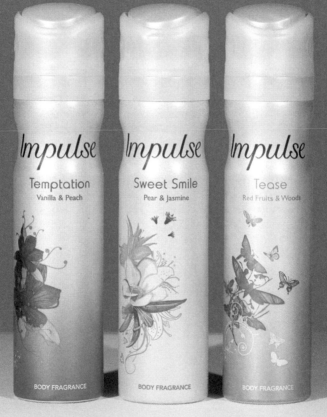

One could never accuse 1980s hair of understatement or restraint. During a single sleepover, my girlfriends and I might backcomb our roots, sweep hair into a side ponytail high enough to make our heads tilt to one side as though in permanent sympathy, secure with a gaudy plastic accessory, perhaps pop in some lengths of lace and then, most importantly, crimp it like pie crust before lashing with enough lacquer to stiffen overcooked linguini. No self-respecting adolescent girl was without her own set of crimpers. Mine came from the catalogue, along with most of my possessions, and took an eternity to heat up before plateauing at hotter-than-hellfire. I would then take sections of hair, place them between the corrugated hot plates and close the crimper, clamping hair tightly, then release to find it moulded into frizzy zig-zags à la Cyndi Lauper, Siouxsie Sioux, Kate Bush or Madonna (or so I imagined).

Much more important than this effect was the enlarging capabilities of crimping. They made flat, thin, Anglo-Saxon hair relatively enormous and then (as it is now, in all honesty) mega volume was my ultimate goal. Safety and hair condition were, sadly, much less of a priority. The smell of singeing hair during crimping sessions was not at all unusual, neither was the sight of broken-off hair tips floating tragically down to one's lap as collateral damage in the pursuit of crinkly, oversized barnet. But we didn't care, nor did our parents, who barely noticed that we held deadly weapons in our dressing tables.

Amazingly, it wasn't the advent of Health and Safety and a more litigious culture that saw off the crimping iron, only fashion. Crimping became desperately uncool and our ambitions were gradually redirected towards spiral perms and super-straight layers. Except now, as with every other dreadful style choice of the past, crimped hair has been adopted by hipsters in some knowing nod to post-modernism. And while I do think in the right hands and context (like a catwalk show or seventh birthday party), crimped hair can still look pretty fabulous, I can't deny that modern crimpers – ceramic-plated, heat-regulating, fire-resistant, slimline, adhering to basic life-saving safety regulations – do rather spoil all the fun.

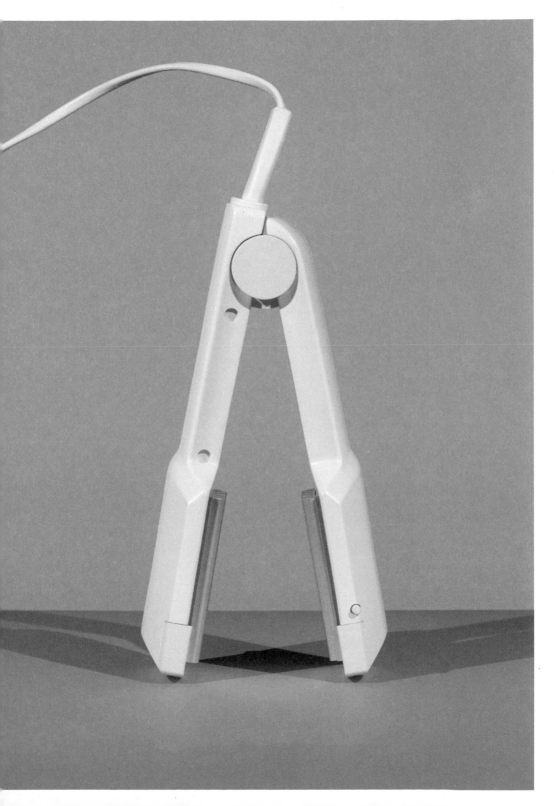

Papier Poudré Blotting Papers

It's ironic and rather pleasing that one of the hottest beauty items of my youth was this, a distinctively elementary invention from 1903. Papier Poudré, little books of oil-absorbing papers, were sold at the Body Shop (back when they sold other people's products) and in the kind of fancy gift boutiques that also stocked linen spray and twelve types of pot-pourri. We loved them because they were about a pound a book, had the sort of soft, vintage-looking packaging that was all the rage at the time (I was very heavily into floral tea dresses and Monet postcards in an Athena clipframe), and specialised in dealing with the curse of teenage existence: grease. When shine struck at school, we'd take out a little book of Papier Poudré (decorated with a French portrait miniature of some grand-looking lady in a powdered wig), tear out a leaf and pat it discreetly on our noses as though we were some delicate maidens from an Austen novel, hoping to elicit an invitation to dance.

Upon launch over a hundred years ago, Papier Poudré was hailed as 'A Triumph of Toilet Science' but in fact it's just absorbent paper made from bamboo and impregnated with a little face powder in one of three shades. As a dry skin sufferer, my own use of Papier Poudré was mainly a pose. But I still believe quite strongly in blotting papers on oilier types. When a build-up of grease causes shine, piling on powder from a puff or sponge can cause blotches, caking and orangeness as the powder reacts with any oil and changes colour. Blotting papers, on the other hand, take more away than they add, absorbing grease before leaving only a trace of face powder. And besides, the one-use nature of papers means there's no chance of hoarding spot-causing bacteria for the next use, making them a more hygienic choice.

I'm not the only one who loves them. At time of writing, blotting papers are enjoying quite the resurgence, with Shiseido, Boscia, NYX, Sephora and others launching their own versions. Even Chanel recently developed their own papers, housed in a chic little black book. But I like Papier Poudré best because not only were they the first, they're also still the prettiest.

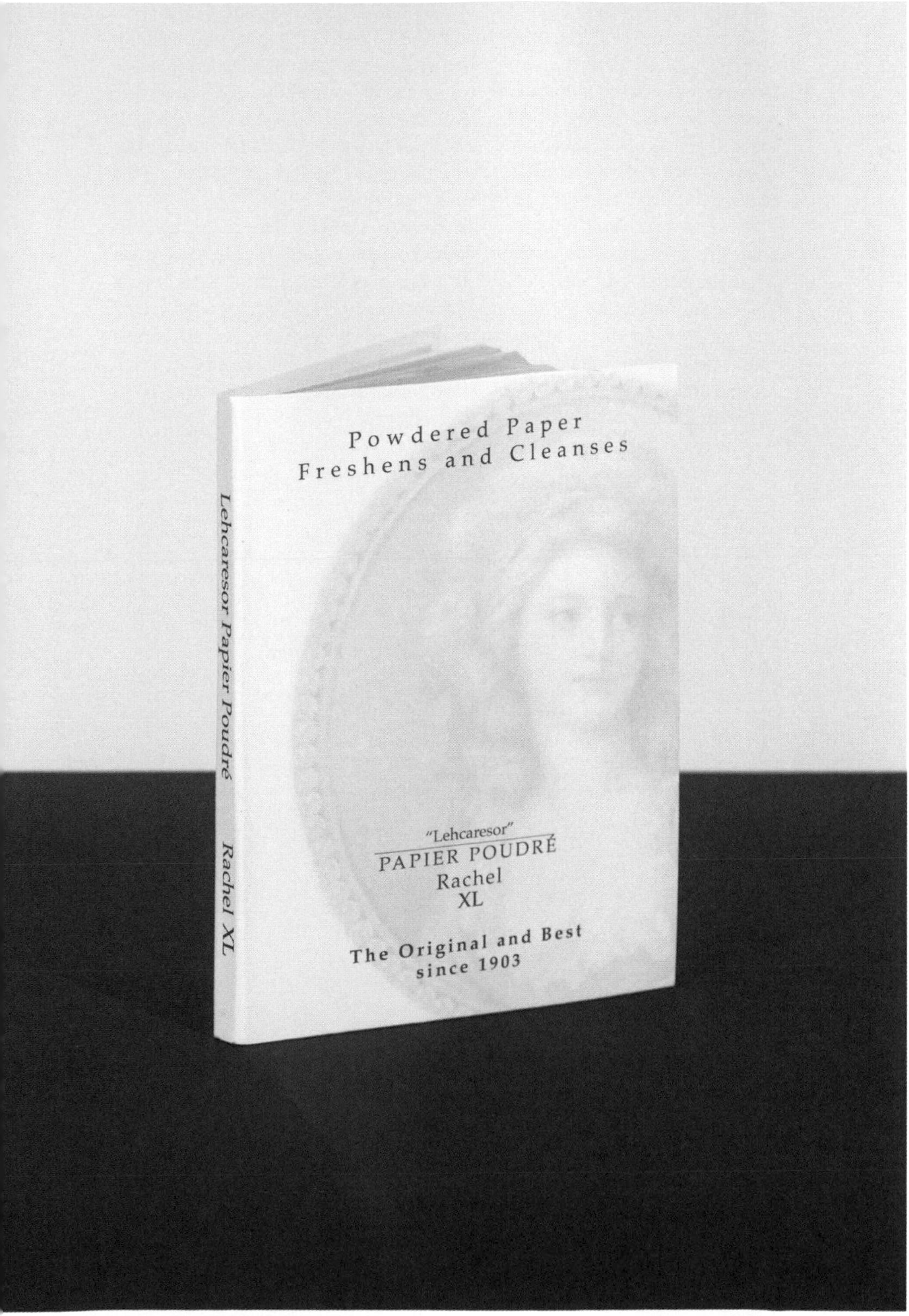

Powdered Paper
Freshens and Cleanses

"Lehcaresor"
PAPIER POUDRÉ
Rachel
XL

The Original and Best
since 1903

Lehcaresor Papier Poudré

Rachel XL

Hair mascara, like deely boppers and a Big Yellow Teapot, was just not something I was allowed while growing up, however much I pleaded (curious from parents who encouraged me to taste red wine, read *Rubyfruit Jungle* and watch *The Deer Hunter*, but still). Thus the appeal of these boldly coloured mascaras, bought for peanuts and raked through sections of hair to add streaks of yellow, hot pink and purple, became so acute that I felt as though I might die of uncool without at least one tube to call my own.

Fortunately, a primary school sleepover at Lynda Rees's house allowed some illicit streaking and hair to colour-co-ordinate with my C&A cerise ski pants and batwing jumper, and her turquoise dungarees and matching bolero. The colour payoff was dreadful, the strands instantly felt as though dredged through syrup and baked in the sun. I had dry, crispy hair behind an apologetic tint of diluted Pepto-Bismol. I was still convincing myself I looked cool when my dad arrived to collect me, glanced at me witheringly and told me I looked like Su Pollard.

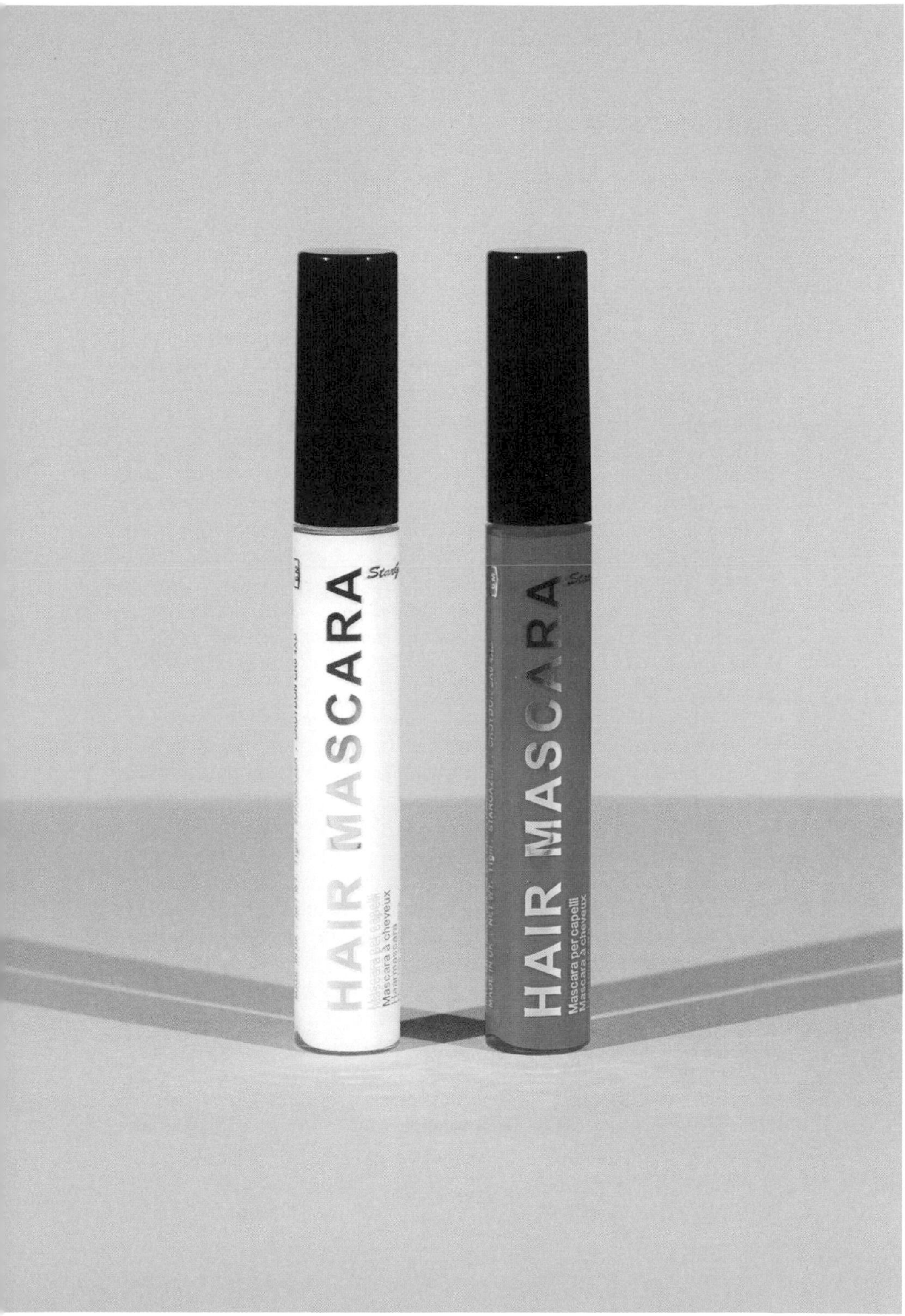
HAIR MASCARA
Mascara per capelli
Mascara à cheveux
HAIR MASCARA
Mascara per capelli
Mascara à cheveux

Did anyone's mum *not* have a set of Carmen rollers in the 1970s? A bulky plastic case of nineteen assorted curlers to be plugged in well in advance of a big night out? For several years, no self-respecting woman with hair below their ears was without them. One merely had to switch on, wait for the case's metal rods to heat up the spiky rollers around them (an interminable period of time by today's standards), then when ready, take the appropriate-sized roller (the smaller the Carmen, the tighter the curl) and wind a section of dry hair around it, up to the scalp, securing with a U-shaped pin, and allow to cool.

It sounds like a fiddly and convoluted process now, when we're accustomed to digital tongs that heat to piping in seconds, but at the dawn of the 1970s Carmens sparked a home haircare revolution that directly shaped the beauty routines of today. Where women had previously had their hair set weekly or fortnightly in a local salon, now they could do it themselves before work. Styles became softer, curls more relaxed. A woman could now change her hairstyle from straight to wavy to curly on a daily basis.

The concept of rollers themselves was nothing new – women had been winding hair around something resembling modern rollers as far back as ancient Egypt – but the ability to heat them electrically, rather than leave rags or curlers in overnight, represented a huge advance. And while Carmen wasn't the innovator (Panasonic made the first set of heated rollers for the Japanese market), its rollers were the most loved, due to their extraordinary reliability and robustness. In 2011 Carmen owner Russell Hobbs was contacted by Sue Peel, a nursery officer from West Yorkshire, who assured the company she'd been using the same set of Carmens every day since 1971 and they were still nobly curling her hair a treat.

Her loyalty to the brand is fairly typical. The world's greatest session stylists wouldn't dream of turning up for a *Vogue* cover shoot without a box of Carmens in tow. Whenever I guest on daytime television or the news, I invariably find that the make-up artists (always by far the most interesting and fun people on set) keep a set of Carmens (or Carmen impostors; it's true that the name Carmen is used for all spiky rollers in the same way 'Hoover' is synonymous with vacuum cleaners) hidden away like a shopkeeper hiding dirty mags below counter. They bring them out because, unlike tongs, which add uneven heat to the hair, and modern digital rollers, which heat fast but fall out easily, or velcros, which add body but no curl, Carmen-style spiked rollers shape the hair into even curls (small rollers) or big, smooth body (larger ones) that lasts.

And they shouldn't be confined to the pros either. If you think rollers require too much skill, you couldn't be further from the truth. Truly, these are the hair tool for people who can't blow dry. You just wind them into rough-dried hair quickly and fairly haphazardly, allow to cool while you put on your make-up, then remove to reveal big, bouncy volume. And if further persuasion were needed, I am of the unwavering belief that everyone looks more glamorous and more beautiful when sporting a head full of cooling Carmens. It's a fabulous look and just too Old Hollywood to resist.

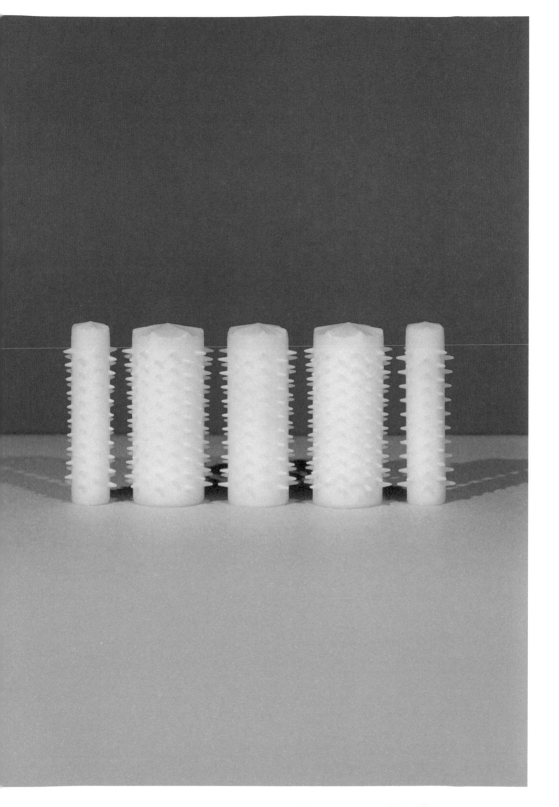

No beauty brand sums up the 1980s as succinctly as L'Oréal Studio Line. This was an inexpensive styling range designed to shape your hair in 'any way you like it', housed in covetable packaging inspired by Mondrian's primary coloured squares and black lines, marketed via TV adverts starring a troupe of male and female models with upwards of three different but equally preposterous hairstyles on each single head, all tearing onto set through backdrop paper. If this weren't already eighties enough for you, then came a male model miming a saxophone break, while a girl with a gravity-defying hairstyle sings into a vintage-style Shure microphone. The whole thing was so absurdly brilliant and iconic that French and Saunders parodied the Studio Line by L'Oréal campaign in one of their legendary Christmas specials, renaming the range 'Stupid Line, by Not Real' (look it up on YouTube, it's marvellous).

But Studio Line was only barely a case of style over substance. Yes, the powerful and targeted branding meant we teenagers wanted primarily to be seen with the designer packaging, but the products within were actually pretty great. A cut above regular high street fare, Studio Line's Styling Cream was hugely popular with the cooler boys at school, while Shaping Gloss, which smelled overwhelmingly of furniture polish and never quite washed off hands, was the only product for arranging your messy bob in a perfect state of Madonna dishevelment. The Studio Line image was so strong and of its time that, inevitably, it couldn't quite make the transition into the twenty-first century. It's now called Studio Pro, packaged in serious black and yellow and represented by mega models such as Xiao Wen Ju and Karlie Kloss, all thick hipster eyeliner and studded leather. The products are still very good, but unlike its previous incarnation, Studio Pro is unmemorable.

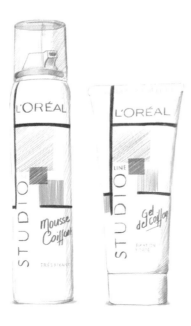

Bath pearls were little, gelatinous and translucent bubbles containing Body Shop perfume and bath oils. You'd drop a couple under running water, and the bubble would dissolve, releasing fragrant, skin-softening goodness into the water. The novelty and prettiness of bath pearls, combined with their impressive, pocket-money-friendly price point of 10p for a luxury bath, caught the public's imagination, and Body Shop couldn't shift them fast enough. Sensing a good thing, Boots, M&S and the rest of the high street followed suit with heart-shaped bubbles, star-shaped bubbles, bath pearls for kids, foaming bath pearls, pearlescent, clear, marbled, boxed, jarred and every other conceivable variation, and everyone received bath pearls for the next two Christmases, regardless of whether or not they even bathed.

Bath pearls became the pot-pourri of the late eighties and early nineties, filling up little bowls and displayed in guest bathrooms, like piles of gemstones or salmon roe. In the end they were so ubiquitous, and so ripped off by companies who didn't really care what they put in them – even if it was base-quality cooking oil made to reek of air freshener and sold in pound shops – that gradually bath pearls became irretrievably naff and we all moved on.

Sadly, I'm sure the attractive appearance that made bath pearls so popular at least in part inspired the introduction some years later of microbeads, those tiny, thoroughly useless bubbles suspended in face wash, shower gel and exfoliators, contributing nothing purposeful but to cause grave and lasting harm to our environment. It's a terrible shame, because in more innocent times bath pearls were rather jolly and good.

I remember my first leg shave like I remember my first period. The former was much worse. I'd been rifling through my mother's products for something to steal, as usual, when I came across my stepfather's razor. I was barely 12 and had paid zero attention to the perfectly acceptable hairs on my legs and yet I suddenly felt an overwhelming urge to shave them all off. I promptly sat on the bathroom carpet (yes, really. The eighties were peculiar) and shaved my bone-dry legs, so entirely without lubrication that the razor sort of chugg-chugged down the skin as I dragged it, like Blu Tack on glass. Satisfied with my handiwork, and smug that I'd avoided a single nick when even my dad's chin seemed permanently covered with tiny squares of blood-soaked tissue, I snuck off to bed before anyone saw me. I woke two hours later, not immediately sure whether my legs were actually on fire, or if I'd dreamed it. They were red raw, swollen, bumpy and stinging like nothing I'd ever known. Christmas – and a Philips Ladyshave – couldn't come soon enough.

The first Philips Ladyshave launched in 1950, soon after its male counterpart and four whole years before competitor Braun followed suit. The original Ladyshave was a little white and silver handset with rows of oscillating blades. My own Ladyshave, some thirty-five years later, was the same tomato red as everything else in the eighties – phones, duvet covers, cars in posters – but was otherwise largely unchanged. I absolutely loved it, and I now find myself wondering why no one I know uses one. Ladyshaves are a weirdly underrated form of hair removal. We now expect gadgets to offer something more scientific (like the IPL hair removal technology of Philips' Lumea, for example) than a mere shave and forget that this one actually offers heaps of advantages over an old-fashioned blade.

For one thing, an electric shave can be taken anywhere and used in a hurry, where a bath or shower is impractical. For another, it doesn't shave off fake tan, which blades do, leaving colour streaky and uneven (though admittedly, by the same token, blades exfoliate dead skin well). An electric is painless, rarely causes bumps on the body, ingrown hairs and other skin annoyances unless skin is extremely sensitive, and it's safe to use in even, erm, delicate areas. A Ladyshave may not be quite as close as a blade and doesn't offer that same borderline orgasmic sensation of perfectly smooth legs against clean sheets, but the modern versions come pretty close. All but the cheapest models are no longer mains or battery operated and they charge in five minutes flat. Why Philips doesn't shout about them is a mystery to me.

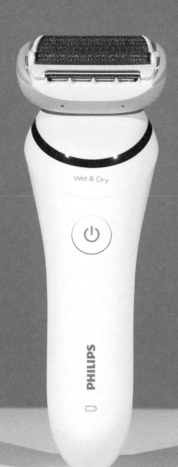

Depending on your age, you probably either believe Tweed perfume is as resolutely 1970s as the spacehopper, or as much a beacon of the 1980s as Annie Lennox's leather gloves.

In truth, even if you remember the flat-top from the first time round, you may not be as old as Lenthéric's big seller, which was actually launched way back in the 1930s. Knowing the perfume has been around that long slightly takes the curse off a brand that hindsight might otherwise judge a little harshly. 'Tweedy' has come to suggest hardy, stoic and outdoorsy – none of which are hugely attractive qualities in a sophisticated lady's fragrance. Vintage ads for Tweed by Lenthéric, though, suggest associations with a confident, Parisian elegance rather than a rural magistrate, joylessly judging a funniest parsnip contest at the village fête. In the 1950s, in fact, Tweed ran a competition with a first prize of a fortnight in Paris, a $6,000 fur coat and $500 spending money. Entrants had to complete the limerick: When a fragrance is perfectly right/You can wear it both morning and night/All products marked Tweed/Are just what you need/… Entry forms were to be sprayed or sprinkled with Tweed hairspray, shampoo, cologne or powder as a proof of purchase, thus presumably putting whoever had to open all the envelopes off the stuff for life.

If, either side of the war, Tweed's appeal was as a safe choice of first scent for a demure young lady, then by the seventies and eighties the scent's customers had grown up with it, and its sights seemed squarely set on Refined Mum. Its popularity was in part down to the way it conferred cosy class, but was cheap enough for frequent discreet spritzing without concerns about the cost of replacement. It was, it has to be said, a cheap perfume attempting to sell working-class women what it imagined they aspired to. Now, the brand fully played up to the whiff of the bucolic about its name. In one memorable commercial, Beethoven's Pastoral symphony played over scenes of a country church wedding and in 1990 Lenthéric launched Tweed Country Collection, with an ad voiced by telly vet Christopher Timothy. It couldn't say 'rural old money' any more clearly if it came with a brace of pheasant and an ill-advised affair with the stable lad.

The scent itself worked with the image. Tweed is a mossy, floral fragrance built on a bosky quality that might variously be described as 'resinous' or 'decaying wood', depending on how charitable is the wearer. And wearers there certainly still are, for while Tweed's heyday may have long passed, the fragrance is still available to elegant nans and those who crave a bit of retro familiarity. I was excited to revisit it for this book, then terribly sad to find it gave me a five-hour headache.

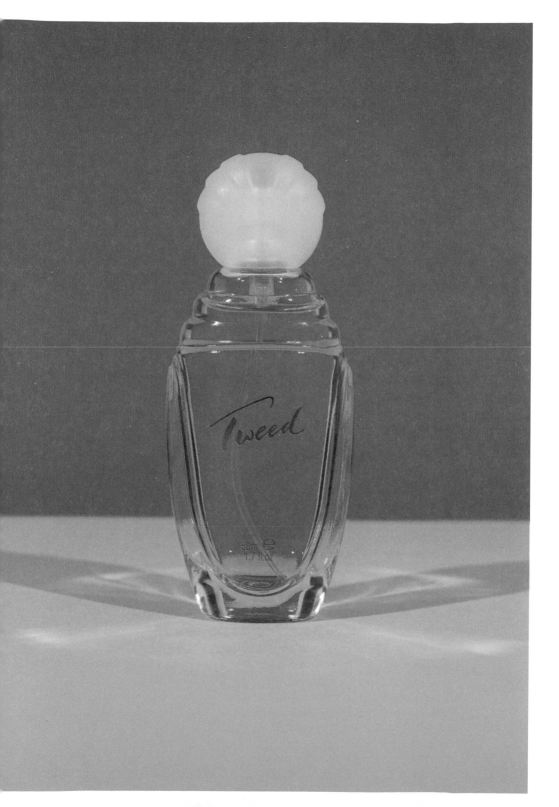

I'm asked frequently at events which make-up brand is my all-time favourite. It's an impossible one to answer given that no one brand is equally brilliant at everything. Knowing your beauty brands is about knowing where each excels and what to cherry-pick from whose product line. Just as one might choose a telly from Sony but an amplifier from Cambridge when shopping for a home entertainment system, one might buy a powder blush from Nars, a mascara from Lancôme, a brush from MAC, a bronzer from Guerlain and so on. But I realise this isn't a neat answer and so if pushed to commit to just one brand that has excited me most, inspired me most, given me the greatest enjoyment and pleasure in my life, I think I'd have to say this. Miss Selfridge Kiss and Make Up is a brand that, for me, ticked every box.

Sold on a dedicated counter in Miss Selfridge stores (the Cardiff counter was staffed by the most incredible-looking redhead pin-up type, with hair down to her bottom, which rather added to the appeal), this was an extremely well-curated selection of make-up, all packaged gorgeously in white, with a hot pink logo and the odd smattering of kiss prints. It was targeted at teens and students, of course, but it didn't patronise them with only daft, fun colours any more than it bored them with the classics. It was bold and cool, rarely faddy, always wearable. I couldn't get enough. Miss Selfridge's Doris Karloff was my very first red lipstick – a matte, true pillar-box crimson – and together with my vintage Levi's, Smiths T-shirts and Dr Marten shoes, we had a ball. Copperknockers, a metallic coppery brown that in hindsight made me look like dead mackerel but was nonetheless present for my first snog, was so popular at my school it was practically uniform. Maiden Over was a peachy-pink blush I wore with a wash of Bit Sweet orange eyeshadow, to which my English teacher Mrs Shakespeare (yes, really) took such grave exception I was held back after class and issued a hundred lines, and the translucent compact was the first time I knew the ladylike joy of powdering my nose.

Kiss and Make Up wasn't flawless, however: I once bought a bath and body set (stamped in teddy bears as well as kiss prints) in the sale that smelled so strongly of wee I began to suspect tampering by a disgruntled employee, and the make-up packaging routinely cracked and split. But it was affordable beauty (costing more than Rimmel and Miners, less than Revlon and Max Factor) that never seemed like a consolation prize to those who couldn't afford luxury. It was hugely desirable in its own right, and went on to inspire Next to launch its own (excellent, now dead) make-up line, as well as those elsewhere on the high street.

In the 1990s Kiss and Make Up was relaunched and woefully repackaged in matte black and silver and, for the first time, it blended into a crowd of generic budget brands, and was soon discontinued for ever. Sort of. In 2006, as part of their fortieth birthday celebrations, Miss Selfridge released some limited edition palettes, each containing legendary items from the original Kiss and Make Up line. The fact that I was by then so sunken by postnatal depression that I failed to buy some, causes me actual bodily pain. And so if you did, and could live without it, I hereby offer a lifetime of free babysitting, lawnmowing and a bottomless beauty goodie bag.

Wella Shockwaves was the first time I'd ever seen a haircare brand marketed at my friends and me, with apparently zero regard for tedious adults. Here were lurid-coloured styling products in transparent tubes covered in edgy graphics, all promising to create hairstyles our parents wouldn't be seen dead in. Unarguably, Shockwaves hair gels were the star turns. There was Strong Hold, a yellow gel used to fashion hair into spikes, make flicky fringes stand aloft, or to define the tracks left by hair comb accessories worn at the temples (we'd sometimes squeeze it directly onto the comb, like paste on a toothbrush). Wet Look, a pinky-blue gel, existed purely to make hair appear sodden. Default application consisted of smothering over soaking just-washed hair, thus denying it the opportunity to dry properly. The result was shiny, stringy curls and locks that gave everyone the impression you'd either just had PE or been plunged head first into a flushing lavatory (not uncommon). Then, quite literally, came the fallout. The gel, having finally dried to a crackle, would flake away at the slightest move and sprinkle itself over your school uniform.

The smell of both formulations was identical: sticky, chemical, utterly delicious. It wafted from the backseats of school buses, down the snogging couples-packed corridors of discos and pierced through the fug of damp sock in the changing rooms. The modern-day Shockwaves products are a more polished affair – still cheap but better quality and catering for a wider array of looks. I can no longer identify the distinctive Shockwaves smell, but I also wonder if it's there, an olfactory dog whistle, detectable only by sixth form and below.

Mum, launched in 1888 ostensibly to prolong the life of the expensive silk stockings of the time by restricting sweat, was the world's first deodorant and on that basis alone it could legitimately claim its iconic status. But the revolution really began in 1952, when female inventor Helen Barnett designed for Mum the first ever roll-on applicator. Inspired by the invention of the ballpoint pen four years earlier, Barnett fitted a large plastic ball around the mouth of the Mum bottle which, when pressed against the surface of the underarm, released a small amount of the deodorising lotion to be rolled over the skin. The design was a massive success but quite unwittingly offered yet more benefits to its female users. To cut to the chase, Mum's ergonomic shape and rounded plastic cap became a makeshift masturbation aid to women and girls worldwide. I'd like to claim this discovery as that of my own generation, but a quick Google search proves otherwise. The Mum legacy of deonanism has been passed silently from generation to generation since the time our great-grandmothers were alive.

There are many reasons to love Mum, of course. It remains a very good product, despite having been consistently neglected and repeatedly sold on from company to company for the past few decades. Barnett's ingenious design was to influence countless modern beauty packaging concepts, from eye serum to lip gloss. Mum introduced an environmentally sound alternative to CFC-emitting aerosols and made the roll-on the world's preferred deodorant type. The planet has much to thank it for. But so, too, do multiple generations of women who were once sweaty, bored teenagers with a raging libido in need of release.

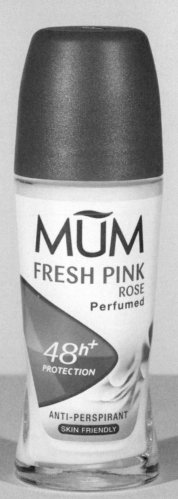

A pointy-bottled medicated shampoo marketed aggressively at families, Vosene seemed to live on the side of the bath in every one of my school friends' houses, though not in mine (my old, single and boarding school-educated father had, shall we say, a relaxed relationship with hygiene; we barely had hot water). Launched in 1949 to clear family dandruff and deter nits, Vosene contained a host of unpronounceable chemicals and perfumes that gave it the brutal aroma of Izal loo paper soaked in floor disinfectant (it has recently been reintroduced with a modern and entirely different formula). And yet still, for my entire childhood, I coveted Vosene, or perhaps more generally, fetishised the kind of normal, wholesome British family who shampooed with it. It was only during the research for this book that I found its once familiar early eighties TV commercial, and in it the narrative subtext of the Vosene mum having been secretly rogered and impregnated by the milkman. Forty years of familial shame began to trickle down the plughole.

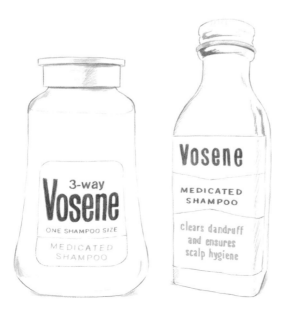

At the risk of sounding 300 years old, I see schoolgirls nowadays and am each time blown away by how much older and more sophisticated they seem in comparison to those in my day. To a generational outsider, they seem so swooshy of hair, so white of tooth, so bedecked in Jack Wills. By contrast, my friends and I were a ramshackle bunch – all bad highlights, customised clothes from the market and schoolbags that came free on the cover of *Just Seventeen*. To us, style and sophistication weren't instinctive, they were literally sprayed on from a bottle of Body Shop White Musk. It's surely no coincidence that my entire upper school of hormonal girls sought to smell of something extracted from the glands of a scrotum, albeit that of a male musk deer and crucially, in the case of Body Shop, not a real one. Unlike the cruelly obtained real thing, synthetic musk harmed not a soul but smelled almost as filthy. As well as this, the largely unchanged formula contains warm, rich vanilla, and the heady scent of lilies, rose and iris – a potent cocktail that, when sold at an excellent price point, makes for a worldwide bestseller.

Body Shop has so many contenders for iconic status, of course. The phenomenon that is Mango Body Butter, for one. Early products it should never have let go, such as Raspberry Ripple Bathing Bubbles, Milk Bath, Colourings Mascara, Pineapple Face Wash and the Orange Bath Oil I once poured down the sink in order to fill the bottle with vodka to take on a residential school trip (it tasted like loo cleaner). The Body Shop philosophy is as iconic as its products. The early adoption of recycling, sustainability and free trade initiatives, its revolutionary campaign against animal testing that inspired many other brands to take their cruelty-free ideals and better them. But I think Body Shop (it has dropped the 'The' since being acquired by L'Oréal) would probably say White Musk is the product for which it is best known. And despite not being a huge fan myself, I'm rather comforted to hear from the unfeasibly sophisticated teens I know, that White Musk is as popular as it was in my youth. It's a good, solid, affordable scent, if not as wholesome as some parents might like.

I once heard Dolly Parton say that she'd grown up idolising the hookers of her small town in the mountains. Where others saw gauche, she saw glamour; where they saw brassy and cheap, she saw beauty, defiance, inspiration. And it recently struck me that this, in essence, is how I feel about Dior's Poison.

Born in 1985, Poison emerged screaming at the top of its lungs to great controversy and extraordinary success. This was a huge, all-encompassing scent that announced itself from a hundred yards away, affording its wearer the gravitas of having kicked her way into a crowded saloon, gun cocked, ready to deal with anything she found there. People were quick to voice their disdain and mockery, but for several years Poison continued to dominate. For a young girl in a small town who felt weird, other, bullied and teased, Poison yelled of another world, where sheer strength of personality was more important than politeness, modesty or class.

I was sleeping over at a school friend's house one night and saw a tiny bottle of Poison – one of those sold in a set of five mini fragrances at airports – on the bathroom shelf. I asked if I could smell it. My friend's mother said I could have it, given that her husband felt embarrassed whenever she wore it. A few weeks earlier, I had stayed at the same house and seen said husband give his wife a state-of-the-art Rowenta iron for her birthday and these two events were instantly and inextricably linked in my mind.

I loved Poison's demands to be noticed and its ability to annoy the kind of men who preferred their women to blend in. It's not polite, it's whorish, and it positively revels in the fact. I still have a great deal of admiration for perfumes that don't mess about and for the women who choose to wear them, and so feel quite sad about the devaluation of Poison. Its brute force and ubiquity in the 1980s have made it the victim of both changing fashions and outright snobbery. It is unfairly grouped with other 1980s power scents like Giorgio Beverly Hills, Passion and Paris (when in fact it's much closer to Frédéric Malle's wonderful and revered Portrait of a Lady), and so my heart sinks when I see Poison standing next to a load of insipid celebrity fragrances in a Superdrug locked cabinet, like a lobotomised hellcat in a cage. It is woefully undeserved.

When sprayed judiciously (and you really do only need the tiniest amount), Poison is actually rather gorgeous. A powerful blend of coriander, plums and berries that smell as though steeped in hard liquor, big, blowsy flowers like rose, tuberose and jasmine, it's a big, overripe, juicy scent – a walk of shame in an apple-shaped bottle. I rarely wear it but keep a bottle in the house for the occasional day when I just don't give a damn.

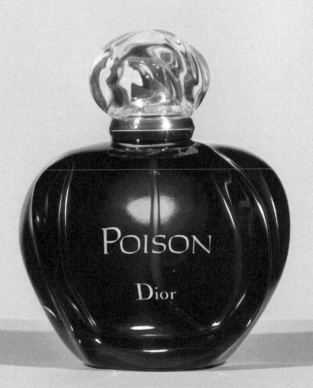

There is no product more quintessentially teenage than a Lip Smacker, the inexpensive, sweet-flavoured lip balm sticks launched in 1973 in the US and still residing in school pencil cases and backpacks the world over. The balms – sold at a rate of 25,000 per day – come in hundreds of flavours and limited editions, and range from classics like raspberry, mango and watermelon, to brand names like Skittles, Chupa Chups and Coke, to bizarre and somewhat gag-causing flavours like Maple Bacon, Hamburger and Sweet Potato Fries. But it all began with a strawberry.

Former CEO Jess Bell decided his glossy lip balm needed to be different, and more fun than the rest. The balms of the time either tasted of their active ingredients – camphor, beeswax, generic masking fragrances – or of nothing at all, and so he set his lab to work on a fruity-flavoured balm. This one simple, commonsensical decision makes Lip Smackers arguably one of the world's most influential beauty brands, in that the vast majority of lip balms that came after it were designed to taste if not of foodstuffs, then at least of something pleasant. Forty years since its launch, Lip Smackers is a juggernaut of a brand. They are distributed widely and cheaply without sacrificing any desirability, and sourced by collectors so devoted to the flavoured lip balm cause that they will pay hundreds of dollars for a rare Lip Smacker flavour on eBay.

For American teens, they remain the default balm for softening chapped lips, but on this side of the Atlantic they feel alien. The gaudy, cheerful packaging seems thrillingly foreign, like something I'd pick up in a New York drugstore, and this is no doubt part of their appeal to British children. But to me, they always felt like an accessory to a life only seen on TV imports: a balm for the students of Beverly Hills, 90210, Degrassi Junior or Sweet Valley High, for kids with brace-straightened teeth, who knew how Dr Pepper and root beer tasted, who called icing 'frosting' and jam 'jelly'. I felt simply unqualified to wear it.

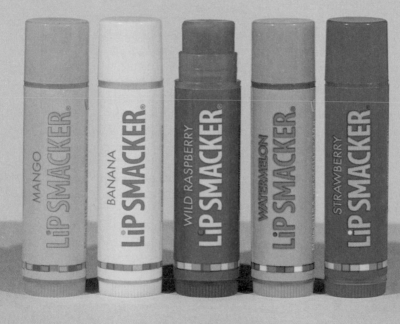

Charlie is an extremely important perfume and few realise it, possibly because of its low price point of around a fiver and its now slightly downmarket positioning. But when launched by Revlon in 1973, this revolutionary beauty icon was marketed less as a fragrance, more as a lifestyle accessory for the modern, emancipated career woman. Charlie expressed this generational shift in several important and groundbreaking ways. An early Charlie campaign was the first ever fragrance advertising to feature a woman of colour (first, African-American model and businesswomen Naomi Sims, and, later, Darnella Thomas); another was the first in which models wore trousers (a style the brand kept for almost all future advertising); and another, highly controversial, campaign depicted a sexually assertive businesswoman (or lech, depending on your perspective) patting a male colleague on the behind – a tongue-in-cheek comment on the sexual harassment women had endured in the workplace for decades.

Even as a child, I could tell that Charlie was doing something differently. The Charlie woman, always healthy, confident-looking and happy, seemed aspirational in a way the Impulse girl, hanging around waiting to be swept off her feet by a man with a bunch of carnations, just didn't. Instead of posing gracefully, goddess-like, before studio lights, the Charlie model was always outside, striding purposefully and cheerfully out of frame as though she barely had time to pause for the click. Even Charlie's name played deliberately with gender expectations, and it was implicit in the brand's marketing that this was a scent to be bought by women for themselves, with their own money.

The scent itself (a chypre – unusual for a cheapy, but wholly fitting in this case) was, inevitably, no girlie cliché. A warm, outdoorsy, fruity floral at first whiff, it dried down into something a little more masculine – a herbal, woody, musky blend that in its original form was rather magnificent. I'm delighted to see Charlie regain its street cred and amass a new cult audience in recent years because its core values are as relevant as ever. And the perfume, while now reformulated and certainly not what it was, is still rather pleasant and cheering to see on the shelf.

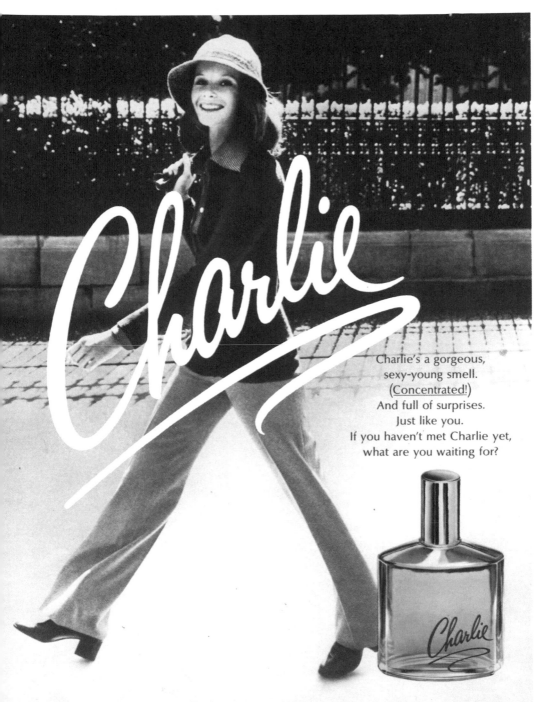

Charlie's a gorgeous,
sexy-young smell.
(Concentrated!)
And full of surprises.
Just like you.
If you haven't met Charlie yet,
what are you waiting for?

A most original fragrance. By REVLON

For an entire decade, there was no greater desire than that of a teenage girl for a spiral perm. Evenly ringleted, romantic, effortlessly natural-looking and entirely frizz-free, this was some kind of follicular nirvana that would undoubtedly pull at least one, if not all three, members of Bros. It was years later, after the worst perm since records began and countless other disasters, before I realised that the problem with spiral perms is that they only existed in magazines. I understood all too late that they were actually the work not of perming lotion and rollers, but of professional session stylists with a set of good barrel tongs.

This knowledge, if acquired when it mattered, would surely have saved me a load of pocket money spent on boxes of Poly Papilloten. This, while not a permanent wave, was a chemist-bought kit comprising a couple of dozen bendy foam rods and a styling spray, promising to mimic the effects of the magical spiral perm that seemed not to exist. You sprayed sections of hair, wound each around a neon-pink rod, then bent it back on itself, much like a croissant. When the whole head had been wound, and resembled an exposed brain, you retired to bed to allow Papilloten to work their magic, while dreaming of hair like Neneh Cherry's. Each time, without fail, you rose from your pit able to meet at least one of the requirements to join Def Leppard.

It seems unimaginable now, when hair products take up aisles and aisles in chemists and supermarkets, that prior to the late 1980s most shampoos and conditioners for European hair (with the exception of dandruff shampoos) were pretty generic: the former, a washing-up liquid with floral scent; the latter, fabric softener by any other name. Both were used by entire households, regardless as to whether a coarse-haired redhead, baby-fine blonde and over-processed poodle perm were all living under the same roof. Those that did aim higher tended to market matching duos of shampoo and conditioner that 'worked together' to improve a single hair complaint, such as dryness.

Enter Salon Selectives by fancy-seeming foreign haircare brand Helene Curtis, with a more tailored approach and a television ad campaign with super-soft rock jingle that gave every impression of having been made up after the recording had commenced. Salon Selectives featured four non-sequentially numbered shampoos and four lettered conditioners, each targeted at specific hair concerns, to be mixed and matched at will. Wet-look hair gel building up on your roots and drying out your ends? You needed shampoo 8 for a deep clean, and conditioner P for protection, and so on. For a couple of years, we bought into it in droves, and the influence of this mix and match approach can be seen throughout the industry.

But from my point of view at least, Salon Selectives will always remind me less of shiny, bouncy tresses, more of the time in my teens when I became so drunk at a Smash Hits Poll Winners after-party that I unwittingly pulled a boyband member and ended up lying fully clothed in a bath, wearing odd shoes and clutching a bottle of wine, singing the Salon Selectives jingle (the catchiest since Bodyform sanitary towels') at full pelt. Truly, there is no moment in my life, however calamitous and depraved, in which however few brain cells are functioning, when I am not on some level thinking about beauty.

For me, there are three publications that signify the start of the festive season: the Argos Catalogue, the double issue of the *Radio Times*, and the Boots Christmas Gift Catalogue. Each is best accessorised with hot mince pies, cold double cream and a variety pack of coloured Sharpies, ready to encircle items and plot one's Christmas shopping list/festive viewing schedule/letter to Father Christmas. I can't remember a Christmas that didn't include these key rituals, nor a time when Boots didn't hold huge appeal. It's easily one of my all-time favourite shops and I still visit frequently, to buy Dove deodorant, Gillette razor blades, Colgate toothpaste, Neutrogena body lotion and all the other everyday toiletries not sent by brands. Friends who've moved to Australia, America and the Continent tell me that as much as they miss Tetley Tea, Heinz Baked Beans and Marmite, what really leaves a hole is the absence of Boots the Chemist (my expat friend Jason calls Boots the 'forty quid shop', since it's seemingly impossible to spend any less per trip). As much as I love a foreign chemist myself, I think I would feel similarly bereft and ask, at the very least, that friends airmailed me the Christmas brochure.

It's a veritable porn mag for beauty lovers. Soap & Glory hampers of shower cream, bath foam and body butter, variety packs of Seventeen flavoured lip glosses or two dozen No7 eyeshadows in a palette resembling a Farrow & Ball paint chart. Soap on a rope for the dad, some grooming collection stored inexplicably in a china mug, perfumed coffrets for husbands clean out of ideas. There are a small handful of career achievements that are disproportionately important to me because they speak directly to my childhood and teenage insecurities or passions. They include seeing my face in the Selfridges Oxford Street window, addressing the Oxford Union and writing a one-off column for the Boots Christmas magazine. I like to kid myself that some teenager, curled up on a sofa and pretending to do her homework, circled one of my recommendations in felt-tip pen.

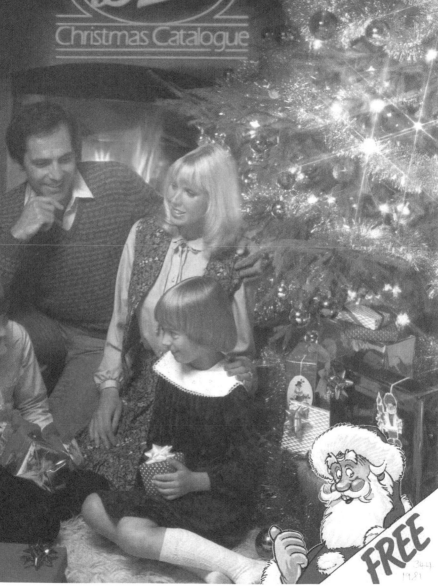

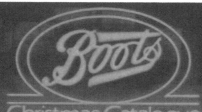

Boots
Christmas Catalogue

FREE

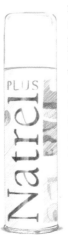

In the mid-1980s Britain was obsessed with natural beauty. The Body Shop, by now the coolest, most desirable brand on the high street, had almost single-handedly changed the beauty landscape and suddenly the ambiguously perfumed petroleum-derived products we'd always used unquestioningly were replaced by those containing essential oils, fruity fragrances, natural extracts of jojoba, henna, chamomile, shea butter, banana, aloe, rosemary – anything perceived to have come from the ground and not from the laboratory via some innocent bunnies and beagles. Even my nan – a committed user of Max Factor, Cyclax, Yardley and No7 – was suddenly rubbing her tired feet in peppermint foot lotion, and replacing the Imperial Leather with some glycerin bar containing satsuma oil.

Inevitably, everyone wanted a piece of the action and some made more effort to uphold Body Shop quality and principles than others. Boots' response came in the form of Natural Collection, an affordable range selling shamelessly Body Shop-inspired but nonetheless cheerful and rather nice fruity bath foams, lip balms, body lotions and other skincare. A natural haircare brand named Henara went from niche health stores to supermarket aisles, and at the upper end of the market, a wonderful little apothecary in Covent Garden's Neal's Yard, selling entirely natural, cruelty-free products in beautiful blue glass bottles, finally found the audience, recognition and buzz it deserved. But for every Neal's Yard Remedies (now an international brand, still made here in the UK) there was some soulless multinational chasing the natural fad for some easy shareholder dollar. By the time we reached 1990, one could seemingly shove a leaf or daisy on a bottle of toilet bleach, spend a packet on marketing, and people would immediately consider it more natural than, and therefore superior to, the rest.

I choose Natrel Plus here because, while it was a perfectly good product (there are plenty of disgruntled users mourning its demise on the Internet, many of them claiming quite plausibly that it was the only antiperspirant not to aggravate their sensitive skin), to me, it sort of represents the moment natural beauty became a bit of a nonsense. Here was an aerosol antiperspirant much like any other, setting itself apart with a not entirely honest name, the addition of 'plant extracts', a posh font and some illustrations of the rainforest, plus adverts featuring beautiful people wearing nothing but body paint and loincloth. While the naked models leapt about the tropical rainforest set, the voiceover repeatedly told us this was a deodorant that worked *with* our bodies, not against them. No explanations were given, no further details revealed. By then we neither wanted nor needed them. They had us at 'Natrel'. Like every sweaty teen at school, I collected all the fragrances until I had a line-up of aerosol cans on my dressing table. And quite the eco-defending sophisticate I felt, too.

Like many children of the seventies, and teens of the eighties and nineties, my love life is indebted to Lipcote, the lipstick fixer that kept one's Miss Selfridge lippy fast, however much rampant snogging attempted to topple it. It was painted on like clear nail polish over lip colour, tasted about as pleasant, then left to dry ahead of the school disco. Suitors, faced with the very real possibility of a snog leading to a furtive squeeze beneath Tammy Girl AA-cup bra, were wholly undeterred by its revolting flavour, and proceeded without reservation. A very happy time was had by all. Lipcote – still very much alive and well and nobly facilitating British teenage fantasies – is not the loveliest treat for skin, it has to be said. It tingles a bit and with too regular use dries out the lips. But it's an honest, effective, affordable and wholly optimistic preparation without which my young life might have been infinitely less fun.

Constance Carroll make-up was, for me, a bit like children's ITV, salad cream and vacuuming – we just didn't have it in the house. It was one of the rare brands that despite great popularity and wide availability seemed to exist outside my world. I saw it elsewhere, of course. Constance Carroll was sold very inexpensively in bargain bins and wicker baskets in street markets (where I shopped a lot), early branches of Superdrug (then, a much less polished affair than now: think Aldi to Boots' Sainsbury's) and 'make-up parties' – informal gatherings of school mums, drinking Lambrini and chatting while shopping for eyeshadow in a friend's living room, to which I would have killed my cat for an invitation.

Constance Carroll's simple and popular USP was that it was cheap and wearable. Shades were muted, unambitious, suitable for busy women making up for the office or school gate. Packaging was flimsy plastic with few concessions to desirability or even a vague pretence of luxury. This meant that for years I instinctively associated Constance Carroll with the sight of a cracked eyeshadow or blusher, coloured dust coating everything in the make-up bag of a school friend's mum or stranger on the bus. But there was an honesty and integrity about Constance Carroll and for many years it was the go-to brand for women on a budget who, unconcerned with fashion trends, simply wanted decent, easy, flattering make-up that didn't make a show of itself.

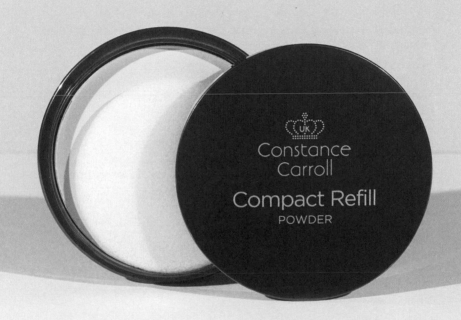

The Life of a Girls' World

Little girl of the 1970s/1980s longs for Girls' World toy, a plastic head with flowing blonde hair, sold with selection of beauty accessories, products and tools.

Santa delivers Girls' World.

Child squeals in giddy excitement for all the many hairstyles and make-up looks she'll now create.

Child plays happily with Girls' World for 1–28 days, learning to braid, applying hair accessories, getting spiky rollers tangled in nylon hair, realising that nylon hair cannot actually be curled without either heat or chemicals, of which there are none in the box.

Child colours strands of Girls' World's hair with the special pens. Younger sibling is inspired to do the same, using paint.

Child applies the included make-up to Girls' World's plastic face, realises that it's practically invisible and feels unpleasantly like chalk on a blackboard, opts to use Biro instead.

Child turns handle on Girls' World to release hair extension. Piece of Lego/ eraser shaped like hamburger/other foreign body jams mechanism. Girls' World now has insane-looking protrusion of hair five inches longer than rest, which has become matted and sticky from orange squash.

Child decides new hair can be salvaged by cutting in a fringe. Child takes kitchen scissors and cuts fringe at least three inches too short. Fringe resembles floor scrubbing brush. Child instantly regrets.

Child puts vandalised and violated Girls' World in box for next ten years. Parent takes to charity shop.

Child is 40 and longs for a Girls' World.

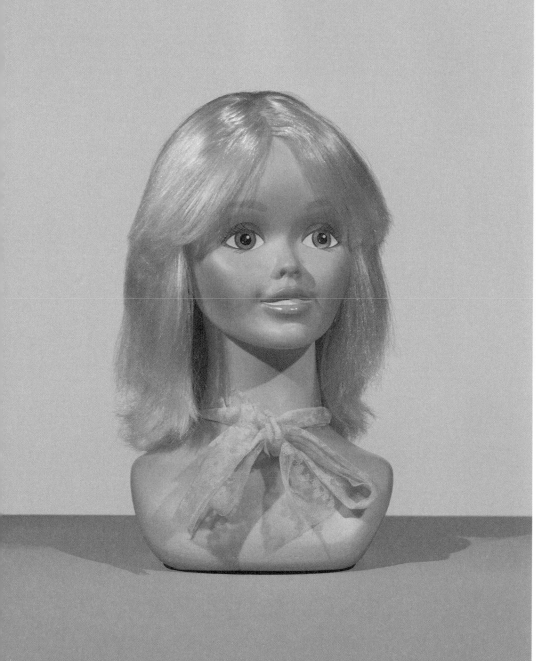

At time of writing, it is some thirty-five years since I saw my first colour change lipsticks, lined up in my local chemist in shades of snot green, egg-yolk yellow and metallic pewter, and in 2016 I'm faintly horrified to find beauty still flogging this wholly stupid concept not so much like a dead horse, more like one that's been embalmed, rested, cremated and scattered, its estate divvied up and bank accounts closed. The idea is that while a lipstick or cheek colour may look wholly unwearable in its package, on application it will, in fact, adapt with the skin's natural pH to create a 'bespoke' pink which, to my eye at least, seems to be an identically unflattering shade of fuchsia, regardless of the wearer's race, colouring or environment.

My question as a child was, as it is now, why? What is the point of pretending to be a revolting green when you are a rather pathetic pink? Why not just buy a pink balm, stick or gloss that actually suits you when it goes on, instead of needing 'developing time' to transfer into something you may not much like? Why would someone have so little faith in their ability to choose a lipstick that they'd like their body temperature and skin chemistry to do it for them? Why does anyone look to a beauty company for these pranks and gimmicks? I remain baffled. I could at least tolerate colour adaptive lipsticks when a fun novelty costing a couple of quid in a 1980s gift shop, but when we are talking about the Diors, Zelens, MACs and Poppy King Lipstick Queens of the world, I do find myself thinking, Grow up.

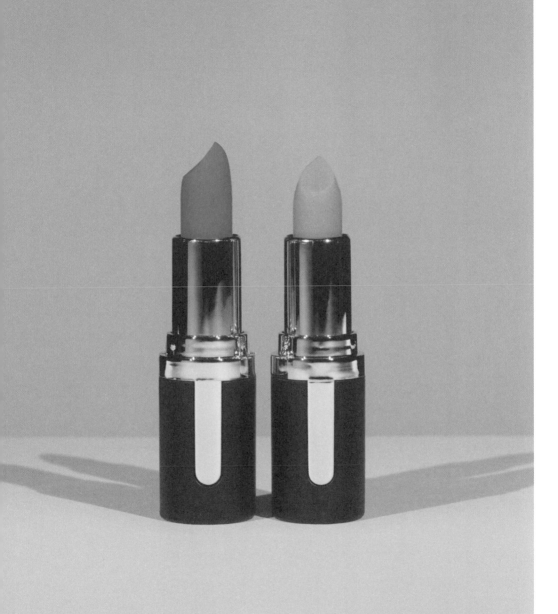

Sun-in was such an irresistibly great idea. Pump the £1.50 spray into freshly washed hair, comb through, blast with a dryer. The heat will activate the Sun-in and hair will emerge brightened, sunkissed and effortlessly golden, like a Californian surfer girl's. But did this actually happen to anyone? Because I recall no such transformation, only that of brown hair turning a permanent shade of tan surely not desired by anyone, anywhere; and of parents returning home from work and clipping their teenagers across their newly Sun-in'd heads. There were no such disasters for me – I chose instead to suffer the indignity of sitting in a salon window, uniform strands of hair being crochet-hooked through a giant head-condom, to be daubed in stinky bleach. But I did once spray Sun-in on my eldest brother, who wanted to emulate David Bowie's hair in the 'Blue Jean' video. Desperate to try it on anyone but myself, I selfishly agreed, and promptly turned him the colour of a Cavalier King Charles Spaniel.

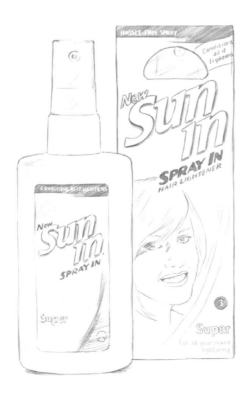

Circa 1986, Boots introduced to the British high street the then radical concept of colour correcting. The intriguing idea was that No7's new green foundation would neutralise any red blotches or ruddiness, leaving behind an evenly toned complexion. Sold on the innovation but frustrated at the idea of a new type of beauty product I couldn't adequately test on myself, I went with my red-cheeked school friend Zillah to get some. I'll cut to the chase: she looked like she'd been plunged face first into a vat of pistachio ice cream. No amount of blending could blur the streaks, nor lessen the chalkiness. She practically glowed in the dark. After so much enthusiastic purchasing, it must surely have seen the lowest repeat-purchase rate in Boots' history. Still, it was a true trailblazer. Colour correctors now sit fully within the beauty mainstream and a generation of women is learning to apply them properly. Props to No7 for nobly pushing us through the pain barrier.

Sachets seemed incredibly modern and exciting in the eighties. Overnight, it seemed, service stations dispensed ketchup and mustard in them, beauty brands filled them with shampoo or face cream and glued them to the pages of magazines, and one-use products – like face masks from St Ives, deep conditioners from Linco Beer and Vo5 – emerged as the new way to try beauty products with minimum financial outlay. The most popular of these among kids and teens were Shaders & Toners, a collection of foil-wrapped, one-use, wash-in/wash-out hair colourants costing less than a quid each. They were hugely appealing to us young people because one could simply forgo a couple of Mars Bars and a pack of Bazooka gum and instead get some plum, copper or mahogany hair to debut at school on Monday, and, crucially, their theoretically ephemeral effects meant one need not seek parental consent before taking the plunge.

The fly in the ointment came when the popularity of both Shaders & Toners and frosty highlights (applied with a perforated rubber bald cap and hook), collided to fairly catastrophic ends. Shaders & Toners had, it turned out, a Dr Jekyll and Mr Hyde level of duality. If the hair was natural, then the Shaders & Toners dye was about as noticeable as a dove in a blizzard. But if it had been highlighted, as ours so often had, then it penetrated deeply, turning hair a sort of rust-orange or the tone of a blueberry milkshake for the next three months at least. One by one, pupils bought a sachet and jumped off a cliff, like Thomas Hardy's flock, each learning nothing from the fate of the last, until half my middle school looked like members of a sinister cult. Thankfully, and unusually, I was not one of them. I was too busy attempting to grow out a shaggy-permed mullet to throw yet more petrol on the bonfire.

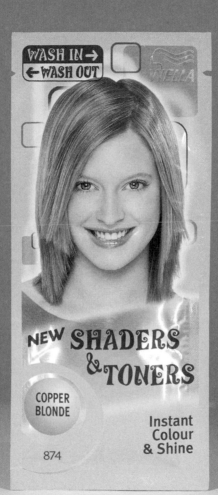

The act of buying an adolescent's first proper perfume is something of a ritual among the upper middle classes of France. When a girl (or boy) comes of age, she is taken to the very grand Guerlain boutique at 68 Champs Élysées, Paris, to select a scent to become her signature, then perhaps on for some lunch or dinner to celebrate. I've always been enchanted by the idea of this unimaginably elegant rite de passage, while still being thoroughly satisfied with my own, less graceful, introduction to the world of fine perfumery.

I had not yet reached my teens when my mother one day returned from a French wine tasting and booze cruise. She and my Auntie Ursula wobbled, giggling, into the house and presented me with a little white textured paper bag, tied with black and white houndstooth ribbon. Inside was a gift-wrapped bottle of Dior's Miss Dior Eau de Toilette. I had not been lusting after it – I hadn't even heard of it – but was instantly enchanted by the ridged glass atomiser and sophisticated, slightly alien fragrance that was more like a men's cologne than the perfumes I'd grown up smelling. In hindsight, Miss Dior was the perfect first perfume, because it was so elegant, ladylike and unlike any of the sugary, girlie scents I encountered over the next few years. It was strong but polite, floral but sharp, romantic but not corny. It refined my palate before I'd really begun – which isn't to suggest I didn't enjoy myself thoroughly during the Loulou/Dewberry/Benetton Colors era, but it did mean that I toyed with those perfumes like casual partners, rather than mistaking them for true love.

By contrast, Miss Dior made me fall irredeemably for chypre fragrances (warm, dry perfumes, almost always built around an accord of oakmoss, patchouli, labdanum and bergamot), and this fragrance family has been easily my favourite ever since. Miss Dior led me to chypres like Chanel's 31 Rue Cambon, Pour Monsieur and No 19; Clinique Aromatics Elixir; Guerlain's Mitsouko; Diptyque Philosykos; Estée Lauder's Knowing; and many more of my all-time most beloved scents.

Sadly, the original 1947 Miss Dior was reformulated in 2005 to conform with new ingredient restrictions. The fragrance Parfums Christian Dior now calls Miss Dior is actually what was formerly known as Miss Dior Chérie, and really doesn't deserve the association (besides, this game of musical chairs is needlessly convoluted to the point of absurd). To confuse matters further, my own Miss Dior has since been resurrected as Miss Dior Originale. It's not quite the masterpiece the 1947 version is, but they still have much in common and both are scents of rare beauty. I feel terribly lucky to have known them both.

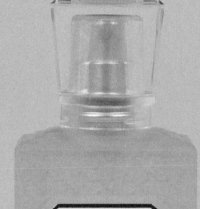

I'm in the wildly privileged position of seeing almost every new beauty product arrive by courier at my house, in huge Jiffy bags, for no financial outlay. It is an extraordinary thing I never, ever take for granted and on the rare occasion I become exasperated by the overwhelming and hugely space-consuming volume of bottles, jars, tubs and tubes I must store and test, I quickly check myself with memories of Body Shop Lip Balm. When this waxy lip softener, costing £1.30, launched in the late 1980s, it was all my heart desired. I would go to Cardiff on the train, loiter in the shop, sniffing the three 'flavours' – Apricot, Kiwi Fruit and the wildly exotic-seeming Morello Cherry – cheerfully considering which I'd buy with my pocket money. Eventually, I went for Morello, and its deliciously sweet and sour taste was rarely away from my lips for the next five years.

It established my criteria for all future lip balms: too shiny and they feel like gloss; too tasteless and I feel short-changed. I want flavour, but not so much that it's like spending the day struggling through a knickerbocker glory. I want balm thick enough to heal chapped lips with only a couple of applications per day, but not so dense that it doesn't spread softly, or turns my lips that horrible chalky white. I want a balm I can wear blended with lip liner on a casual day, but that will also sit under proper lippy without the colour creeping up to my sinuses. I want nice packaging – a tube with a flat, not rounded, spreading surface, a stick with a well-shaped nib, or a pot not so deep that I'm still scraping balm out of my fingernail at bedtime. The Body Shop's Morello Cherry Lip Balm delivered on every requirement but the last and I'm at a loss as to why it's been discontinued.

But more significant than the formula itself was what my pot of Body Shop Lip Balm represented. I think – before I'd ever saved up for my first Clarins cleanser or Clinique Clarifying Lotion – Morello Cherry was the first beauty product I'd ever bought for myself, and was all the more meaningful for it. It represented a financial sacrifice, but also a giddy thrill I'd never previously known. It's the exact same feeling I get now, decades later, when I open my Jiffy bags. I strongly believe that anyone who doesn't feel it, or who has long since stopped, or who doesn't know how it feels to agonise over parting with a sum of money for a single product, or who hasn't later felt elated or crushed with their purchase, or who doesn't at least inwardly squeal when holding a new Chanel lipstick, basically has no business encouraging readers to spend their hard-earned cash on beauty. It's the Morello Cherry Lip Balm effect, and if I ever lose it, I'll know it's time to quit.

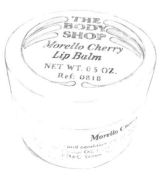

In the early 1990s clear mascara swept both the nation and our lashes while simultaneously being about as much use as a chocolate fireguard. But this didn't matter, because for a generation of comprehensive schoolgirls clear mascara was a means of tiny rebellion against the establishment. The presence of this – let's face it – watered-down hair gel in a mascara tube may have been wholly imperceptible to teachers, boys, parents, anyone with eyes, but we always knew it was there. This, if only in name, was proper make-up bought from grown-up Boots counters (Leichner or No17 were favourites), and chucked in our Chelsea Girl backpacks for topping up on the move (much like the fabled emperor might have carried an invisible cloak in case he became chilly under his new clothes).

Reapplying our transparent mascara during lunchbreak was my first beauty bonding ritual with girls my own age. We'd line up at the too-small basins in the girls' loos, wiggling our clear mascara wands and lacquering our bobbed haircuts into something vaguely resembling Bananarama's, while we gossiped nineteen to the dozen about who'd flirted with whom on the morning bus. Then off we'd go to class, our dress code infringement a delicious secret between us. This tiny revolution was tough on my allowance: every tube of clear mascara became so revoltingly cloudy and full of teenage grease, bits of hair and Cornsilk face powder that it was practically unusable in three weeks flat.

I must grudgingly concede that while clear mascara barely impacted my lashes, it did somehow leave its mark on my life. I still buy cheap clear mascara now, only to tame, groom and fix eyebrows. It's nowhere near as exciting to use as it was back then, but at least it has finally found its calling.

One of my earliest beauty memories is of being pushed around Woolworths, when my babysitter stopped the buggy, unzipped my anorak, and hid inside it a can of Silvikrin hairspray almost as big as me. Up the zip went again, the can's lid jammed against my throat, and out we sped onto Blackwood High Street. It was impossible for Silvikrin to ever live up to that first heady experience, but nevertheless it's a marvellous product I see constantly on professional photo shoots and frequently reach for myself. It has a stronger hold than Elnett and is less 'wet', making it a great choice for up-dos that demand less flexibility than, say, beachy waves. It's also still very cheap – if not quite a steal.

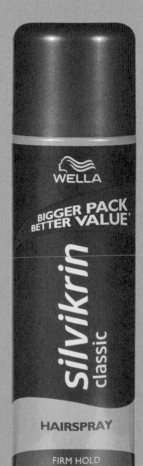

Giorgio Beverly Hills arrived in Britain during the 1980s glamour soap era of *Dynasty* and *Dallas*, with their heroines in shoulder pads, huge statement clip-on earrings, satin turbans, sparking up their Sobranies with desktop cigarette lighters made from onyx and marble. This almost traumatically potent scent, from a designer few British people had even heard of, seemed exactly the kind of thing Alexis Carrington Colby or Sue Ellen Ewing might wear en route to irrevocably mess up someone's life. Giorgio Beverly Hills, born from an expensive Melrose boutique of the same name, was exactly right for an era that celebrated, if not delivered, wealth, success and conspicuous consumption for all. Along with Dior Poison, it became a worldwide phenomenon, scenting everyone and everything within a fifty-yard radius of the Giorgio Beverly Hills woman. Consequently, it was famously banned by several Los Angeles restaurants, whose clientele had begun to complain of food and dining rooms tainted with perfume.

Sadly, no such ban existed in the South Wales valleys, and my mother, having picked up the yellow and white candy-stripe box of Giorgio in a ferry terminal, sprayed it liberally and with impunity. I thought I could gag no more, until the day she threw her handbag into the back of her Mini and unknowingly smashed the Giorgio Beverly Hills bottle on the car floor. Out it seeped, into the carpet and soft furnishings it marched like an unstoppable rebel force, permanently diffusing the entire car with the stench of stale gin. Thereafter, we travelled in rain or shine with every window down, and my head dangling in the breeze, gasping, cursing and longing for the 80s to end.

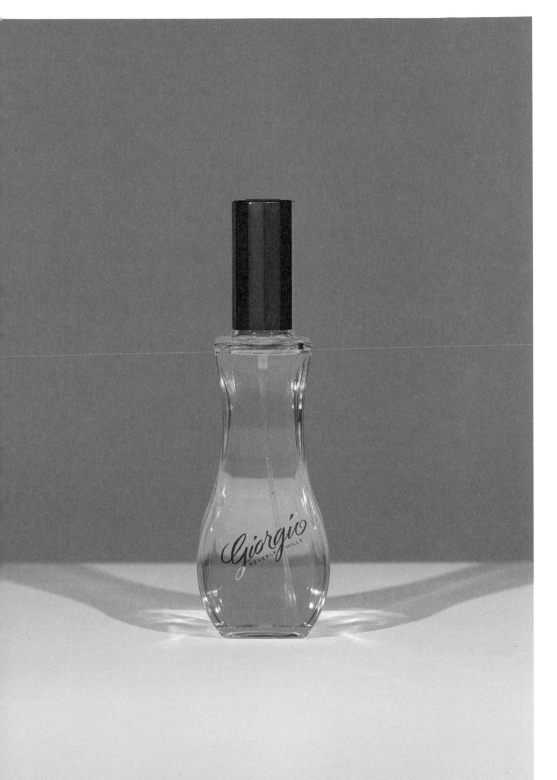

It's hard to imagine it now, but pre-1995 almost all mainstream nail polishes were versions of pink, red, peach or beige. A few market-stall neons worn by goths, punks and other alternative style tribes notwithstanding, there were few of the blues, greens, oranges, greys and black polishes we now think nothing of wearing to a wedding or job interview.

Then came young US medical student Dineh Mohajer, who, frustrated at not being able to find a polish to match her favourite sandals, mixed up her own lacquer in chalky, opaque baby blue from her tiny college dorm. The shade was named Sky, the Hard Candy brand was born, and every cool girl – led by nineties icon Alicia Silverstone (who wore Sky on the David Letterman show, causing a run on the polish) – wanted all they could get. Soon, and despite Hard Candy's impossibly thick, gloopy formula (the original was Essie white and cheap salon supply store dark blue, mixed together in a ketchup bottle), fashionable nails were lurid seventies lime, swirly petrol-blue metallic, creamy mocha brown, sparkly bottle green and gunmetal grey. We've never looked back.

But Hard Candy revolutionised beauty beyond merely expanding its colour palette. A trailblazer in the cult beauty movement, Mohajer was among the first to sell beauty as a fashion accessory, cleverly dressing each square bottle with a kitsch plastic-jelly ring around its neck, to be worn next to the matching polish. Instead of naff, traditional shades called Peach Parfait, Oyster and Merlot, Hard Candy polishes had endlessly copied names like Porno, Oedipus and Scam. Ad campaigns were cheeky, edgy and with a feminist-lite subtext. She helped fuel the US nail bar phenomenon in Britain, paved the way for urban, female-led brands like Urban Decay (launched a year later), and was among the first modern companies to enter department store beauty halls with only one product (despite being as poor as a church mouse, I somehow scored £10 bottles of Mint and Ice from a dedicated rack in Liberty on Regent Street).

Hard Candy's existence as a unique, specialist brand was sadly short-lived, as Mohajer – and then her new bankrollers LVMH – branched out to make the first mainstream glitter eyeliner, caffeinated lipsticks and (less successfully) Hard Candy base, eyeshadow palettes and even clothing and cellphones, an over-ambitiousness that within five years had robbed the brand of much of its cool and quality. By then, Dineh had jumped ship (she recently launched a similarly niche nail brand called Smith & Cult), and Hard Candy disappeared into obscurity for many years, until 2009, when it was revived in a somewhat dampened form by US supermarket Walmart. Gone were the cool chunky bottles and hip, no-nonsense logo and font. The new Hard Candy resembled a poor woman's Barry M, lacking the punch, edge and collectability of the original game-changing line.

In 2015, for the twentieth anniversary, Walmart released a retro collector's set of the Hard Candy icons – Sky, Coconut and others – in their original packaging, and sent beauty nerds and eBayers into a frenzy, but this apparently didn't convince decision makers of its long-term viability. This is perhaps a tragedy, because Hard Candy was, without question, a trailblazing, important and extraordinarily creative brand that altered the beauty landscape for ever.

It is one of my more shameful secrets that I used a Buf-Puf cleansing sponge almost every day throughout my teens. Shameful not because Buf-Puf is a bad product (it isn't), but because I was so over-zealous in my exfoliation that I may well have caused lasting damage. My defence is that Buf-Puf was the only thing that could de-flake my then horrendously dry skin, and allow me to apply make-up without bits of skin peeling off in my hands (I literally never went anywhere without one), and besides, I was hardly alone. Buf-Puf launched in the 1960s and was still huge when I hit puberty in the eighties. Advertised as a way to deep-clean pores and prevent and remove blackheads, it was available in disposable single sponges or in a larger, egg-shaped sponge to be changed every few weeks. There was peach for sensitive types, pink for really sensitive types, and hardcore white for everyone else. One lathered up with a face wash, then scrubbed the skin with a damp Buf-Puf before rinsing and applying skincare. It mostly worked a charm, until I'd suffer a particularly bad day at school and take out all the frustrations on my poor face that should rightly have been directed at Robert Anderson and all the other boys who teased me about my dry, flaky skin. I'd know I'd gone too far when applying my moisturiser felt like taking an acid bath, and the skin on my chin would redden and weep.

But as harsh and unappealing as Buf-Puf could be, I do give it credit for leading the movement towards exfoliating with textured materials, rather than textured products – one I still believe in to this day. For the past twenty years, I've used a common-or-garden terry cotton flannel rather than a Buf-Puf, but if you plan to track down the latter (they are no longer available on the high street, but Amazon stocks them – check out the hundreds of evangelical reviews), then I plead with you here to exercise caution when scrubbing and go so, so easy.

There's a rather indelicate saying in the beauty industry, the gist of which is this: 'You can't polish muck, but you can roll it in glitter', meaning that if all else goes wrong with a face of make-up, just whack on a load of sparkle and you've got yourself a look. It works just as well as a metaphor for life. A little frivolity and glamour can make almost any crap day at least a little cheerier and I think if I were to sum up this entire philosophy in one beauty product, I'd choose Barry M's Dazzle Dust. I've been using this cheap, cheerful, cruelty-free and British-made brand since childhood and I still hold it in the deepest affection.

It began over fifty years ago, when 16-year-old entrepreneur Barry Mero began flogging wholesale hair lacquer to the punters on his mum's East End market stall. He quickly turned a profit and expanded into colour cosmetics. Unable to fit his whole name onto the small labels, he shortened his surname to 'M' and paid someone a tenner to design him the logo we still see today. Dazzle Dust, a fine sparkle powder that presses into moisturiser, creme shadow and blusher or sweeps over bare lids, available in many shades (depending on season), was introduced early on and for me remains his hero product.

Dazzle Dust epitomises all that's good about make-up. It's jolly, colourful, heaps of fun and perfect for experimenting with creative looks. It's what I bought with my childhood pocket money (it's still less than a fiver, decades after launching) and it's absolutely true to say that it helped lay the foundations for a lifelong love of mucking about with make-up. I still love glitter and while my beloved MAC and Illamasqua glitters are all well and good (and they really are), to spend fortunes on sparkle is to rather circumvent what makes it so enjoyable. The joy of Barry M is how deeply unpretentious and egalitarian it is. It's for people who love make-up, whether teenage girls, drag queens, clubbers, toddlers at play, or kids dressing up for a school concert. It's a brilliant product and a true beauty icon. Transform your day and go and buy some.

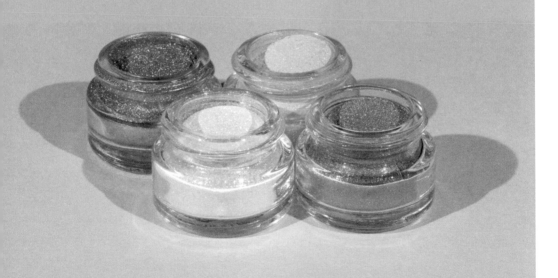

Immac is so unfairly maligned and I'm sure this stems less from what is actually a very good product, more from how thoroughly useless we were in using it as kids. My first foray came when I agreed, with no due reassurance and some implied authority, to remove my school friend Lynda's moustache. We were on a caravan holiday in Tenby and the act of going out to buy the cream behind my father's back felt less like an errand, more like a secret operation. We bought the leg cream (which smelled like fly strips) not the sensitive facial version, smeared on enough to ice a three-tier cake, then removed it only when Lynda was practically weeping from the soreness. She then spent the next five days with an angry red patch signposting exactly where the much less visible 'tache had quietly resided before we'd begun meddling.

Despite the relentless advertising and marketing of Immac at teenage girls, I gave it a swerve for the next decade, my perception skewed by screw-up. I discovered only latterly that when done the right way, Immac (or Veet as it's known in these times of globalisation – booo) does do the job very well. The stinky fumes have long since departed (though there is a bit of a whiff – you wouldn't mistake it for body cream), it doesn't strip skin of moisture and it does remove hair pretty quickly and thoroughly (the opaque formula makes it hard to miss a spot). The reason I don't use it that often is that I actively enjoy shaving my legs (especially as a dry skin sufferer: shaving is a great method of exfoliation) and I can't quite be bothered to go to the hassle and expense (yes, I do have to pay) for what amounts to three days without leg hair.

Where I do think Immac excels is in the treatment of facial and bikini line hair. Most other methods have quite off-putting flaws. For instance, threading the upper lip is agony and often causes spots; waxing face or bikini can suffer the same pitfalls and cause hairs to ingrow. And a razor to the face or ladyparts, just NO. One can laser or IPL, but I am wary, if only when it comes to my face. Immac is a much less complicated proposition. Just pop on the dedicated sensitive skin formula, wait a few minutes, wipe off, rinse. A tube will last ages, too.

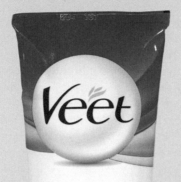

I feel great and enduring love for Rimmel (now Rimmel London), a brand that's managed to remain cool and current from day one. And so I find it rather ironic that Rimmel's most memorable product is not their wonderful Kate Moss collection of mattes and nudes that look as sophisticated and luxe as a department store shade, or the wonderful Instaflawless, a balm for swiftly perfecting the complexion for photography, or the wonderful and affordable brow, lip and kajal pencils, or the thousand other cutting-edge Rimmel products I've worn and loved in my lifetime.

No, Rimmel's greatest icon is the deliciously naff Heather Shimmer lipstick. While this long-lasting frosty purple-mauve deserves our congratulations in managing somehow to combine both brown and silver undertones in one shade (I mean, it's not something I'd think to shoot for, but bravo to them in getting there), but also for its undeniable status as the lip colour of the 1980s. We snuck Heather Shimmer into our school bags, we wore it to discos in the hope of pulling boys, used it to add weight to our fake IDs when attempting to score alcopops in pubs. But more than that, what made Heather Shimmer such a juggernaut of a product was its rare cross-generational appeal. Truly, our grandmothers and mothers were just as likely to wear it as we were, all of us united in our inexplicable desire to look as though dead from hypothermia.

And yet I note with some admiration that the decade never really ended for some. I admire any make-up item that transcends fad to become a classic, soldiering on year after year, ensuring its manufacturers daren't retire it for fear of customer revolt – especially one that does so while being infinitely less cool or even flattering than so many of its contemporaries. Heather Shimmer, rather impressively, is still among Rimmel's bestsellers and for me, spotting it on a twenty-first-century mouth is as satisfying and comforting as finding a surprise double yolker in a box of eggs. I will never again wear it, but I'd be deeply saddened to ever see it go.

Does the word 'bobble' mean anything to anyone under 35? I worry that it doesn't. For the rest of us, bobbles were hair elastics twisted into a figure '8' and clamped in the middle with metal. At each end was a brightly coloured plastic cube or ball, that was fed through the tightly wound elastic loops to secure plaits, ponytails and bunches in place. Bobbles were sold by the pair in chemists and newsagents, on little perforated cards that were torn off a large display, just like Big D pub snacks only without the underlying Page 3 boobs. My father, recently left by his wife, was tasked with doing my hair for school. He was so woefully inept that I spent each morning standing on a chair, listening to him swear as bobbles pinged, snapped and ricocheted, one after the other, out of his hands and against the kitchen wall. Marc Jacobs has often tried to revive the bobble – at both his own Marc label and while at Louis Vuitton – and each time, I've been bemused at the willingness of fashion fans to pay over £100 for something my father was ultimately forced to buy weekly on foolscap from a local cash and carry.

An instantly evocative bath gel smelling of thyme, pine and juniper. Only old-school Radox – and the slightly posher, more European, Badedas – seem to give you that amazing, almost momentarily *painful* hit, as you submerge your cold aching body in a hot foamy bath for a long, relaxing muscle soak. Its huge, chemical bubbles – always stiff enough for the making of beards and the protection of modesty – are strong-smelling and fresh almost to the point of pine toilet cleaner, but just manage to stay on the right side. Not particularly wonderful on dry skin, but still irresistibly blissful and cosying, especially when teamed with a mug of hot tea and the Radio 4 Shipping Forecast.

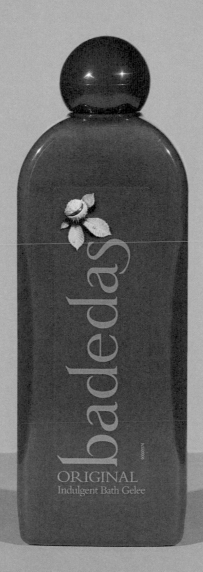

Tinkerbell was make-up for children sold in Woolworths, newsagents and the kind of toyshop you only found in British holiday resorts. Peel-off nail polish, star-shaped stick-on face decals, clear lipstick that barely left a trace on the skin. It was hugely popular in the eighties, but I suppose these days would be seen as an evil akin to asbestos-roofed classrooms and candy cigarettes. I'd share my reminiscences of Tinkerbell, but they would be very much with my nose pressed up against the cake-shop window. To me, Tinkerbell was posh and extravagant. It was owned by the kinds of children who got individual Kellogg's variety boxes of cereal, and whose clothes came from C&A, not from kids they'd never met. I longed for it but never owned a single piece. I suspect it was fortuitous, since I was forced to plunder my mum's make-up bag and learn how to put on the real stuff.

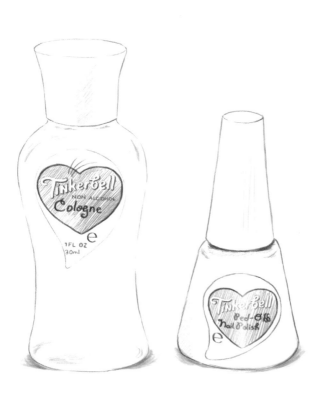

I must disclose that I am broadly unkeen on lip gloss, and my relationship with even those I like has been less one of enduring love, more a sporadic run of booty calls. Sometimes it feels right, like when I'm wearing a very heavy eye look or practically nothing but tinted moisturiser, but I'm never fully committed and am still much more likely to reach for a tinted balm. This is partly because I'm averse to glosses' common texture of soft-set jam smeared across the mouth, trapping hair and grit like flypaper. I think of lip gloss as lipstick for beginners, a gateway drug to the proper stuff, and associate them with teenagers who've yet to cut their teeth and move on to the pure joy of bold, dense, saturated colour.

These wilderness years of my own youth were however served rather pleasingly by this, lip gloss that looked like a tiny glass roll-on deodorant, which dispensed sticky, thin, clear, high-shine gloss over the mouth without the need for a mirror. It gave us wet-look lips like Farrah Fawcett Majors and Christie Brinkley, and, as such, seemed utterly correct with powder-blue lids, too much bronzer and huge, Carmen-rollered hair flicks. On the mouth, it had an almost imperceptible peachy tone, a strong and distinctive taste of undiluted cordial and suntan lotion, and all the longevity of a mayfly. Not that we cared, because the ephemeral effects of the roll-on lip gloss allowed us to reach for it frequently and display it to all, feeling disgustingly smug about owning it and ever so grown up indeed.

THE
FUTURE
ICONS

I always do my utmost to judge a cosmetic on its merits, not its price tag. Prince and pauper products sit side by side in my bathroom cupboard. If I recommend anything particularly pricey (and I try, in all honesty, to avoid it), invariably some casual but vocal readers or tweeters will infer that I ride around all day on a platinum Segway and bathe in unicorn tears, so, if anything, for me to recommend an expensive product, it needs to exponentially outperform a cheaper alternative.

Bioeffect does. Quite simply, I have never known an anti-ageing serum work so quickly, and so noticeably, to improve the look of my skin. Within about five days of first using Bioeffect (alone, after cleansing – no oil or night cream over the top), everything looked smoother, more hydrated. There was yet more improvement within a couple of months. It was one of those pretty rare products that I feel cross about having to abandon in order to get on with my job testing others. Nowadays, I get around the problem by using the Bioeffect 30 Day Treatment as something of a reboot between other serums.

The other reason I've been hesitant in recommending Bioeffect is that its history has not been without controversy, albeit indirect. The EGF in Bioeffect's name stands for 'epidermal growth factor', a so-called cellular activator. Applied to the skin, EGF sends messages to the cells, encouraging the production of collagen and elastin. It's a naturally produced substance that would normally reach the skin from the dermal layer, but when applied topically can accelerate the repair of wounded skin. EGF's revitalising effect on skin made it an attractive prospect for the cosmetics industry and in 2010 Icelandic firm Sif Cosmetics launched Bioeffect EGF Serum to huge domestic success.

EGF, though, does not come without scientific baggage. Due to it encouraging the skin's factory to work harder, it can be kryptonite to anyone suffering from psoriasis, which is caused by the body already over-producing new skin cells. There have also been concerns over the relationship between EGF and cancer, based on EGF's indiscriminate treatment of cells and the risk that it will encourage cancerous or pre-cancerous cells to proliferate as much as healthy ones. It should be made clear, though, that there is no suggestion EGF causes cancer in healthy cells, and besides the cellular activators used in Bioeffect are grown in genetically modified barley and are unrecognisable to cancerous cells. But not all EGF-using brands are able to say the same, so please do your homework.

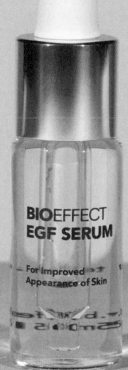

I've received so many tweets, emails and messages over the years from readers who are thrilled to have found this via my numerous recommendations and incessant evangelising. And so I really should give credit where it's due while I have the chance. In the summer of 2009 I was at legendary make-up artist Mary Greenwell's apartment to interview her for a story for *Red* magazine, in which she revealed her favourite products. To cut to the chase: when Mary tells you a foundation is 'divine and exquisite', you listen. So instead of going home afterwards, I diverted to Selfridges purely to try on some Suqqu Cream Foundation, and fell instantly in love.

I've had romantic relationships a fraction as long as my relationship with Suqqu. And while I have been known to play the field with other bases, I know I'll never forsake it entirely.

So for those yet to meet this, one of the greatest foundations on earth, allow me to introduce it. It's a thick, moist, creamy base that is so concentrated it'll probably last you the best part of a year. If you're very oily, you may not like it (it's not at all greasy, but neither is it matte). If you want a sheer, transparent coverage, then there are more suitable products (though one of Suqqu's unique abilities is in mixing exceptionally well with most other things, and so it's terribly easy to either thin it out with moisturiser, or ramp up the coverage of a CC cream by mixing in a dollop of Suqqu). But if you are dry, normal or mature of skin and want a full coverage foundation that will make your face feel as though it's been taken to the opera, look no further. It spreads and blends perfectly, smoothing the skin in dewy, natural-looking light with zero chalkiness or caking. It stays on all day without a single touch-up and furnishes all other make-up with the perfect canvas. But where Suqqu is most extraordinary is in the feel. It has an extremely fine Japanese formula that feels utterly weightless on the skin (if I close my eyes, my face is bare).

It has three notable faults, however: the jar, while satisfyingly weighty on the dressing table, is a complete pain for travel and I normally either decant or leave at home. I also fully understand that sixty-odd quid is an obscene amount of money for a foundation, and the shade range is woefully exclusive, but almost every woman lucky enough to find her match ends up coming back for more, regardless of cost.

And yet this absolutely wonderful base is almost wholly ignored by the company that makes it. It seems pretty unkeen on it, if anything. The counter staff are forever pushing their newer (good, but inferior) foundations like Frame Fix and Dual Effect, often alluding to the possibility that original Cream is not long for this world.

In all honesty, I would no longer despair if Suqqu finally acted on their consultants' constant, low-level threat and discontinued Cream Foundation – though I'd be far from happy. I have stockpiled enough jars to see me through the apocalypse and besides, there are now other bases I love almost as much (Guerlain Parure Gold Fluid, for example. Surratt Surreal Skin, for another) and yet, if I have a big photo shoot or event to attend, I would grab it as instinctively as I would my house keys.

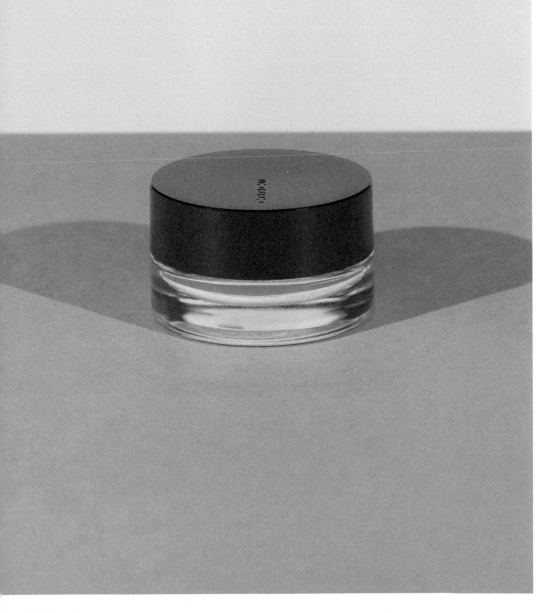

Thanks to the always-on nature of social media, it can feel that we forever need to have our public face ready. If you're someone whose absence from Instagram for more than a couple of hours has worried friends forming search parties, you know how beneficial an instant facial fix can be. But even for those of us not welded to our devices, the rise of one-use masks and intensive treatments, driven in part by influential Korean beauty trends and technologies, has been a godsend. The problem with a lot of pricey face masks and eye serums is that they turn out to be one-use for the wrong reasons; if they're too much faff they just end up gathering dust at the back of the cupboard and ultimately going off (is there anything more frustrating than discovering that an expensive beauty product has died on the vine and now smells of turps? I vote no).

Skyn's eye gels, though, are ideal for the beauty commitment-phobe. While they're by no means the first of their kind, they are in my view the best. You peel off the gel patch (infused with all manner of natural plant extracts, antioxidants and oils, including ginkgo biloba, which I find to be consistently good on dark circles, albeit temporarily), stick under your eyes for around fifteen minutes, peel off carefully and then chuck away. Dark circles are left plumped and brightened, skin firmed, un-puffed and de-crêped. Perfect for a pre-razz pep-up, or for a quick cheer-up when run down, you get eight pairs in a packet, which works out at about three quid a go. They're cruelty-free and ideal for travel too. Holiday selfie onslaught ahoy.

skyn
ICELAND.
Solutions for Stressed Skin

Helps firm and de-puff within minutes

WORKED ALL DAY. STAYED OUT ALL NIGHT. EYES LOOK AS **EXHAUSTED** AS I FEEL... FOUR AND A HALF HOURS OF SLEEP TUESDAY. FIVE HOURS WEDNESDAY. **PUFFY** DOESN'T EVEN BEGIN TO DESCRIBE IT ... **FROWN, SQUINT, FROWN, SQUINT, FROWN, SQUINT.** WHERE DID THESE **DEEP LINES** COME FROM? ... UNDER-EYE AREA NEEDS A SERIOUS INTERVENTION!™

Hydro Cool Firming Eye Gels
WITH HEXAPEPTIDE TECHNOLOGY
Gels Raffermissants pour les Yeux

8 pairs of eye gels | 8 paires de gels pour les yeux
8 x 3.2 g / 8 x .11 oz

Somewhere around 2001 it became completely acceptable to 'clean' one's face without visiting the bathroom, or even lifting one's self from the sofa at all. We already had pre-peeled potatoes, ready-chopped onions, bottled water for those too lazy or precious to walk a few steps to the tap. Now it was beauty's turn to be simultaneously sluttish and wildly cavalier about the planet's general health – not to mention that of our skin. Seemingly overnight, every woman I know began removing her make-up as though wiping a particularly stubborn poo from a newborn's bottom. Chemists' shelves were cleared for pile upon pile of wipes on 3-for-2 deals. Cleanser sales plummeted while landfill rose, and no one's face looked any the better for it.

I admit there are times when wipes are a godsend, of course. Festivals, hospital stays, photo shoots, long-haul flights, evenings when one is too drunk for standing up or exercising even basic dexterity, or when a pre-sex freshen up is desirable. They are essential in removing eye make-up from lids wearing lash extensions (wrap a wipe around the finger and the extensions can be easily avoided) and are always better than nothing at all.

And for all these occasions, I choose these – Britain's bestselling wipes – over any other. They're mild, as thorough as a wipe could hope to be, unsticky, wet enough, not too drying and cheap. It pains me to praise Simple any further, since it is partly responsible for one of the most regrettable consumer trends of all time (though in all fairness, Olay pioneered it via its revolutionary disposable wash cloths in 1999), but I'm encouraged to see so many beauty fans now returning to proper cleansing balm, oil or cream, and seeing dramatic results on their skin. The rise, too, of the micellar lotion (or 'cleansing water') offers something of a halfway house, but it requires cotton wool and so is neither as environmentally friendly, nor anything like as effective, as a good, old-fashioned, washable cotton flannel. It depresses me to tell you that Simple wipes are Britain's bestselling facial skincare product (especially since Simple has so many better products), and I hope one day to be able to discuss wipes like loom bands and the McPizza, but I fear their iconic status is cemented.

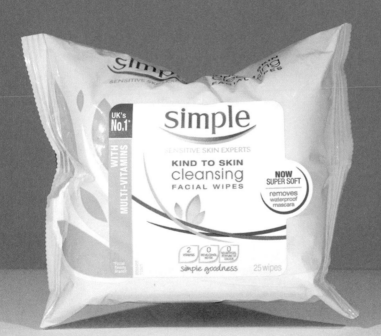

Other false eyelash glues, why do you bother? DUO – sold in Boots, MAC and any professional beauty supply store worth a damn – dries clear, is strong, durable and comes in a proper tube, not some fiddly vial that disappears into your fingernail like a stiletto on a cattle grid. DUO-fixed lashes (provided you trim them to size first – this is an essential step and one that is often ignored) will stay on your lids, not droop sadly onto your cheek. For one 1980s London club night, I even used DUO to glue large, red rhinestone hearts onto the faces of drag queens, and they simply did not budge throughout God knows what level of escapade. Truly, this is the Heinz baked beans of lash glues. Accept no substitutes.

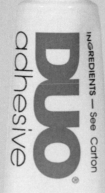

People now seem to be onboard with the idea of a wet hair detangling brush, but I struggle with the popular no-handle designs, which always seem to slip out of my palms when I try to get real purchase. And so while Tangle Teezer, the 2007 invention famously dismissed as pointless on *Dragons' Den* before racking up an annual turnover of £30 million for its British owner Shaun Pulfrey, was undoubtedly the commendable trailblazer, I find this, invented three years later in America, works miles better for me. It cuts through tangles like a hot knife through butter; no drag, no snag, and distributes styling product evenly. I can take it into the shower or bath to brush through a hair mask and it doesn't get mouldy from damp. It even glides through wet hair extensions (which I occasionally employ for thickness – shhhh), and because of the handle can be used with a hot dryer without burning my fingers. Every family should have one. Preferably in leopard print.

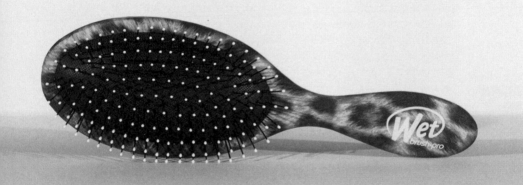

I think Lanolips is the perfect lip balm.

It was created – if the word can even be used seriously about a single ingredient popped in a tube – when founder Kirsten Carriol, dreading the skin-drying effects of the long-haul flight home from her honeymoon, began daydreaming about her childhood holidays on her grandparents' farm. There she was surrounded by lanolin, a natural wax found in sheep's wool. Cosmetics marketer Carriol realised the potential of a lanolin-based beauty brand and, after several years of development, Lanolips was launched in 2009. In the first twelve months, Lanolips sold 1.7 million units.

Now, you may already be turning the page because you're allergic to lanolin. If so, stay your hand. I used to think I was. Lots of us did. Women in their droves still tell me they are. And indeed you might be, but it's much less likely than you think. Due to a misinterpreted study in the 1950s, the risk of lanolin allergy in the general population was hugely overestimated, giving it an enduring bad rep. On top of which, the lanolin used back then was a magnet for impurities like exhaust fumes and pesticides. But progressively tougher legislation and improvements in refinement techniques mean today's lanolin is to the old version as extra virgin olive oil is to the residue in a student flat grill pan. Nowadays, medical-grade lanolin is used to protect nursing mothers and their babies and is even used surgically to treat burns and open wounds. Lanolips goes one further and purifies it even beyond this point.

And it's great on lips. Lanolips isn't shiny but matte. It doesn't mess with your lipstick and send it seeping over the lipline. It's extremely moisturising (I've been known to slather it under my eyes on long-haul flights). And it comes in a massive tube that lives in practically every big make-up artist's kitbag. What more could you ask for? My personal preference is for the exfoliating Lemon Aid version, but the original 101 Ointment is the range's must-have, and not just for the lips. It creates a breathable barrier and can hold up to 400 times its own weight in moisture. An ideal general-purpose emollient, wherever you need one.

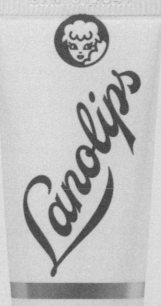

Frédéric Malle is more curator than perfumer. The scents that bear his name are created in collaboration with world-renowned experts, lured with the rare promise of creative freedom. L'Eau d'Hiver, launched in 2003, is the scent of Jean-Claude Ellena, whose day job is as in-house perfumer at Hermès. He created the wonderful Terre d'Hermès (worn by my other half but equally as delicious on women) and further back, YSL's Falling in Love Again and Sisley's Eau de Campagne – all perfumes I admire. But L'Eau d'Hiver is so completely beautiful that I find myself idly sniffing my wrists all day, inhaling so deeply that I fear I'll spirit it clean away.

Yes, as the name suggests, it's warming. But don't mistake that for highly spiced or vanilla-sticky, which couldn't be further from the truth. L'Eau d'Hiver is a much more complex blend of warm and watery heliotrope flowers, almond milk, a tiny whiff of citrus, a pinch of powdery cinnamon and a gentle tipple of booze. This is the gentlest, mellowest, cosiest perfume I've ever had the pleasure of wearing – so transparent, soft and whispery that I expected it to be fleeting, but, to my great delight, it lasts all day (I can still smell it when I lift my toothbrush to my mouth before bed). This perfume is just bliss – like a warm, calming, soothing baby blanket for the nose and yet, very unexpectedly, quietly sexy and deeply elegant. It's clean but never virginal, soft but never girlie, sensual but in no way smutty. It's one of those scents you want to wear all the time, even when alone, because everything seems better when it's nearby.

By the very nature of his operation, Frédéric Malle's scents are reliably distinct, none a passenger among the collection. Carnal Flower, all big, horny tuberose and warm coconut, is gorgeous. The much celebrated Portrait of a Lady, soft, rosy and a bit smutty, is indeed wonderful. Lipstick Rose – smelling exactly as the name suggests – is a playful delight that never fails to make me smile. But of all these exceptional fragrances, L'Eau d'Hiver, to my mind and nose, is the one that will prove truly timeless.

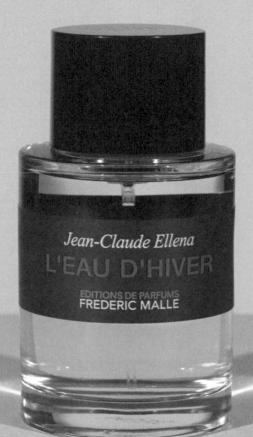

I'm a natural gadget-sceptic. Too often I come across a futuristic lump of plastic that either doesn't do what it claims or does it in a fiddlier way than something a fraction of the price (the myriad cleansing devices when a flannel performs better, for example). But Tria's innovative light, designed to fight acne and serious spots, is no such dust-gatherer – it fights problem skin with impressive pluck.

As the Tria uses non-UV light to kill bacteria, it doesn't irritate the skin – I can vouch for that bit myself. But to put it properly through its paces, shortly after its launch I asked, with some scepticism, two friends to try the device: one had regular breakouts of painful spots; the other had suffered continuously from acne on her chin and lower cheeks for years, and had seen several private dermatologists to little avail. Though dubious, I wanted them to give it a fair, two-month go, but within a fortnight both had reported dramatic improvements to the condition of their skin. The spots had either disappeared or reduced significantly. In fact, the acne sufferer – now completely clear of bad skin and wearing a tinted moisturiser, rather than a mask of thick foundation for the first time in her adult life – made it clear the Tria would need to be prised from her cold, dead hands. 'Only another acne sufferer will understand when I say I'd sooner go without a washing machine or oven than go back,' she told me.

At over £200, the Acne Clearing Blue Light is ostensibly an expensive bit of kit. But for those burdened with acne and severe breakouts, clear skin can be a priceless commodity. For its potential to transform their lives and as a possible alternative to strong medication, I think history will judge Tria's gadget as a bargain.

If eye cream was on Facebook, our relationship status would read: It's complicated. I'm not a believer in eye creams as a necessity in their own right – your current anti-ageing serum and day creams should do a perfectly serviceable job around the eyes and I do believe many women would be better off saving their cash (for what it's worth, I don't even have to pay for eye creams and still, I rarely use one). However, sometimes a face cream will cause irritation or puffiness on sensitive or oily skins, or you might just prefer a lighter texture, and in such cases I certainly wouldn't dig my heels in against use of a specifically eye-designated alternative.

I think the best I've found is Zelens, developed by Dr Marko Lens, a very good plastic surgeon with a particular interest in the eyes. Zelens Eye Cream's mission is to tackle fine lines and wrinkles, dark circles and puffiness, with a wide combination of botanical and high-tech ingredients (as well as oldies and goodies like glycerin) from smoothing sesame protein to Acetyl Octapeptide-3, a 'botox in a jar' substance which is claimed to help prevent wrinkles by inhibiting neurotransmitters which cause the contraction of facial muscles.

Whatever makes Zelens cream work (and it does definitely seem to improve skin texture around the eyes long-term, as well as making them look instantly smoother and more awake. I personally don't buy into any brand's dark circles claims), I'm not the only one to think its results are impressive. I've been in another brand's office when they've had a pot of Zelens Eye Cream on the table, staff with furrowed brows trying to work out the formula like Bletchley Park codebreakers poring over a recovered Enigma machine.

My one reservation, as with so many products rendered unstable by being plonked in a jar, is that the cream should be in an airtight pump instead. Oh, and the price point. It may be enough to make your eyes water.

REN's bestselling, much loved mask, born in 2005, was among the first peels that you could previously only score from a facialist or dermatologist to be made available over the counter. It's a real fruit salad, featuring AHAs derived from passion fruit, lemon, grape and pineapple, along with a papaya enzyme. These last two, in my opinion, are particularly good exfoliants and AHAs in general form part of my cleansing routine about three times a week. They act like a road gang for the face, resurfacing by loosening the bonds that keep dead skin cells in place and promoting growth beneath, leaving a bright, radiant, even skin surface for light to bounce off, giving a healthy, youthful glow. In middle age, I find it's this glow that matters to me infinitely more than the eradication of wrinkles, which don't bother me hugely. Countless conversations with readers suggest I'm not alone in that, and brands are slowly beginning to wise up.

What I like about the Glycolactic Renewal Mask in particular is that unlike some masks and exfoliants, which can be as awkward to remove as Play-Doh from a wool-twist carpet, it comes off easily. It benefits both dry and oily skin, and while it's not for particularly sensitive complexions it's still gentler than a lot of other peels and an unscary option for the relatively inexperienced (my face is like asbestos at this point, and can happily go stronger). I've found it good on blackheads and open pores, and it's got a lovely goopy citric feel and smell. If you've ever fantasised about coating your face in marmalade (we've all been there), it turns out you can go one better.

It's not the only great product from REN, just its most popular and well known. I also love Instant Brightening Beauty Shot, a tightening silicone-based eye treatment that is my pre-party go-to, and the cleansing milks across the brand, which are reliably wonderful.

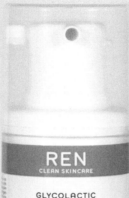

There's something so joyous about a good backcomb. Whether you're attempting a retro Ronnie Spector beehive or a Robert Smith 'lost in the woods for a month' 'do (don't), teasing has always been the best way to get hair to puff out like a pigeon on the pull.

But with a regular brush, the teasing often isn't thorough enough, the effect insufficiently long-lasting. With a comb, meanwhile, the hair can easily get damaged. Backcombing goes against the grain, lifting and loosening the cuticles that grow outwards along the strand (imagine running your fingers up over the ears on a stalk of corn to the tip – and then what would happen if you pushed them down the other way). It's this that gives the hair volume, but in the long term weakens the strands. For volume maximisation and damage limitation, a specialised brush is the way forward.

The excellent Vogetti, thin and draught-excluder-like in appearance, lets you more easily find and tease at the roots. It also sports boar bristles, which naturally condition hair and improve texture. Impressively, you can pick up the Wonder Brush for less than a fiver. A big 'do never came so cheap.

In around 1998, as the 23-year-old junior fashion writer at *Loaded* magazine, I went to see my editor and asked him to allow me to launch a male grooming section in the magazine. Broadly indifferent to anything I did, he agreed a budget of £200 per page all in, and shooed me off without asking what I might do with it. For my first issue, I decided on a hair special. I'd interview Jon Chapman, a session stylist I'd worked with on fashion shoots, and ask him how to achieve a host of iconic hairstyles, good and ridiculous, from Shaun Ryder's bowl cut to Pat Sharp's mullet. I needed product shots to go alongside them and so I picked up the industry contacts book, lifted the phone, and called in my first ever beauty product from a PR.

This, Espa's all-time bestseller, was what arrived a couple of hours later, in a pretty gift bag clutched in the glove of a motorbike courier. And I'm pleased to say it remains a corker. Launched in 1989, it's a deep-conditioning mud mask made from red clay, watercress and apricot kernel oil, that rinses off to leave hair of any type as soft as cashmere with resolutely no grease. I particularly like it combed in after a bedtime bath, wrapped in a towel and rinsed out in the morning, or slathered onto hair on lazy holidays where a slicked-back ponytail is no big deal. But it also doubles as a great body moisturiser, softening rough skin on heels, shins and elbows if you're caught short.

Pink Hair and Scalp Mud never made it into my story, but it did make it into my bathroom. And I have never once picked it up without feeling a fleeting but enormous sense of gratitude for my career, for all the beauty products I'm sent every year, and for the fact that my hair doesn't snap under the strain of testing them.

I was sitting in JFK airport one day, sipping a coffee and waiting for my flight to be called, when a group of teenage girls pitched up at the next table. I began earwigging, as is my wont, and discovered their excited chatter was not about boys, school or TV, but about lip balm. Of course my ears pricked up. Next, each girl produced a brightly coloured little sphere from her bag and unscrewed the top to reveal another, smaller sphere, this one made of solid lip balm. The overall effect was a bit like a mini egg in an egg cup. I was intrigued, and as the girls applied the balm, even though it looked fiddly and inconvenient, I immediately wished I could go back through the gate to the nearest Duane Reade and pick one up. My teen years may be long gone, but I still felt like I was missing out.

I'm not surprised that EOS lip balm spread like wildfire that year. The spark was a Miley Cyrus music video – standing at over 400 million views at time of writing – in which she selects the balm from a table full of them and copiously applies it. Obviously, seeing Miley Cyrus actually putting something on in a video is quite the rarity, as is a shot of her mouth in which her tongue isn't lolling out like a dropped carpet, but this was particularly eye-opening as the product placement is so front and centre in the clip you'd half expect a 'skip ad' button to appear. I have no idea whether Miley was on the payroll or not, but if she was, EOS's investment must have been repaid many times over.

It seems to me that this is a brand that has been launched entirely on the back of celebrity endorsement – whether paid for or free – with Britney, Kim, Christina and a few sundry surname-required celebs queuing up to pose poised with sphere to pout. It's essentially a neat, desirable packaging concept allied to star power, with the quality of the product itself (average) largely an irrelevance. Even a class action brought against EOS for alleged severe allergic reactions (swiftly and amicably resolved) failed to come in like a wrecking ball on the balm's success. A truly modern beauty phenomenon.

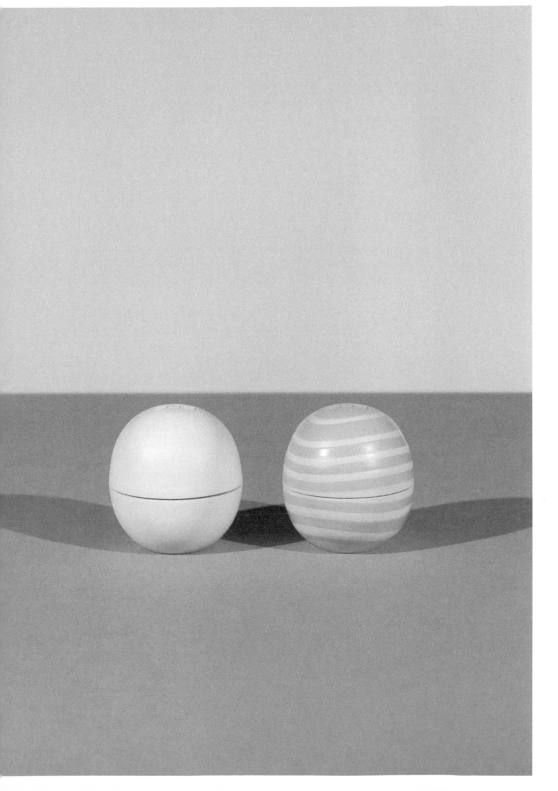

If you ever learned to drive, you may have raised an eyebrow when you were taught that in the event of a skid, you should resist your instinct to turn the wheel away from the direction the car was sliding, and instead steer into the skid. The idea is that by momentarily steering with the skid, the wheels start to turn and you regain control. No, there has not been a mix-up at the printing press, much as I'm tickled by the idea of Jeremy Clarkson's next book featuring a paragraph about moisturiser. The step from this lesson to the treatment of problematically oily or spotty skin is actually a short one. Time and again I see people with these dispiriting problems understandably try to solve them by drying out the skin. But by removing the skin's protective acid mantle and natural lubrication, the result is invariably red, angry and sore. Worse, the confused skin, stripped of natural protection, will squirt out even more grease to compensate.

The way to regain control, counter-intuitive as it may seem, is to moisturise. Mineral oils, shea and cocoa butter and super-rich emollients, I should make it clear, will not help, but the right moisturiser will. Effaclar Duo is the one I've found to have the most consistent results for people with spots. It comes from La Roche-Posay, a brilliant French pharmacy brand that I've found to be extremely reliable and relatively inexpensive. Effaclar contains four active ingredients in a combination designed to treat inflammation, discolouration and the formation of acne marks. It's quickly absorbed and the matte finish will be appreciated by anyone feeling self-conscious about their face's oily shine. While an absolute disaster on my own dry skin, it's the product I recommend most often to oilies and certainly among those most often on the receiving end of glowing reviews from readers.

For severe problem skin, no over-the-counter product is a substitute for seeing your GP, but more often than not, in conjunction with a disciplined cleansing routine, Effaclar proves beneficial and is an excellent first port of call for sufferers wary of steering into the skid.

These days, a truly cult beauty product is a rare thing indeed. Whereas I once had to wait for someone to go to America to score me some Kevyn Aucoin mascara, Carmex lip balm, EOS shave cream or Kate Somerville moisturiser, now I can head to Space NK or specialist beauty magpie stores like Beauty Mart, or even just order direct from Sephora US. The Bioderma micellar and Make Up For Ever palettes and pouches that represented the pinnacle of any trip to France, can now be picked up in Boots, Debenhams or British pro stores like Guru Makeup Emporium; and the Australian friends who once sent me care packages of Lucas's Pawpaw Ointment, Aesop potions and Becca Creme Blush can now save their postage money – I'll just click on Cult Beauty and Amazon and pick them all up, throwing in a few Korean-imported face masks and cushion blushers for good measure.

Getting my hands on these hard-to-find purchases once felt more like pilgrimages, and they consumed me in the most enjoyable and ultimately satisfying way. And while I know I should be pleased that since the e-commerce revolution my life in this regard has become a whole lot easier, I can't help but feel sad the delirious triumph at having obtained a cult product has been replaced by a feeling of deflation that the thrill of the chase has gone.

I mention this admittedly screwed-up mentality, because at time of writing Magic Move remains a true cult beauty find, insofar as it's extremely hard to find in the UK. And that's not the only reason I love it. It happens to be the brilliant Japanese hairstyling pomade used by genius hairstylist Sam McKnight on Michelle Williams in her Louis Vuitton campaign shots (in which she has the perfect hair – big, bleached, effortlessly messy), on the models at the Chanel A/W13 show to add texture and movement to long, smooth hair, and on countless photo shoots since. It can also be used as a brilliantine to grease down and seal split ends, only unlike Dax Wax, Nu Nile and the rest, it's not greasy-looking. And yet nor does it have that horrible, dry-to-touch matte of styling clay that makes hair look so grubby and unhealthy. On hearing about it, I felt that old perverse mixture of frustration and delight that I couldn't easily get it here, and actively turned on by the challenge of getting my paws on a tub (which I did, at Ricky's NYC).

But I know that sooner or later, some UK importer will get wise to its genius and Magic Move will become part of the furniture and lose a little of its sheen, like so many before it, and my eyes will inevitably wander to something less attainable, something more aloof to keep me hanging on. It's pitiful, really. I'm like some immature sap chasing men who play hard to get, desperately dialling their number hundreds of times to no avail, only to go instantly off them when they finally pick up.

Urban Decay's Naked Palette is easily the most famous eye palette in the history of beauty.

I certainly wouldn't have seen that coming when I met founder Wende Zomnir for lunch in 1999. Then, the brand was just launching in the UK and colour was its credo. Urban Decay was all about garish glitters and punky make-up with edgy names. It was brilliant, but nudes were nowhere to be seen.

A decade later and Zomnir and a couple of associates were idly choosing the four neutral eyeshadows they'd each take to a desert island. They threw their selections on a table and, after a little tweaking, the original twelve-shade Naked palette was staring back up at them.

Urban Decay was definitely not the first to make nudes its 'thing' (and when I say 'nudes', I mean all tones naturally present in skin, from milk white to espresso black, from rosy pink to soft ochre and everything in between, not that generic Caucasian shade of buff the industry apparently imagines us all to be). Kevyn Aucoin's Ultima II really invented the modern nudes palette, and Bobbi Brown went on to build an empire from wearable nudes. But I think it's fair to say that Naked inspired most nude palettes that followed – and there have been many.

That first twelve-colour palette, launched in 2010, spawned an empire, including two sequels, a smoky version and an all-over face palette. At one point the brand claimed that someone bought a Naked Palette every five seconds. Today, every beauty blogger owns it. If you're carrying one in your kit you'll always be able to please anyone you make up, and if you have all four, you can pretty much do anything. The pigments are nice and dense, with great colour payoff and blendability.

Not that I'm afraid of colour, but I do generally temper bold flourishes with something neutral – brown, taupe, ivory or chocolate give everything a more sophisticated air and are a particularly good foil for bright lipstick. Neutrals provide the most wearable eye looks by far, ranging from a simple wash of one colour over the lids (using your fingers, if you like), to a more considered blend of pale base, mid-tone eyelid, dark socket and liner, and shimmery, highlighted brow bone. For all this, I personally need no more than four to six shades. Which is why, of all the Naked palettes, the newer offshoots, Naked Basics, are my favourites. These take things back to the original concept, editing out the superfluous in favour of six essential nudes that offer an infinite number of looks, and get around my one nagging problem with multi-palettes: waste.

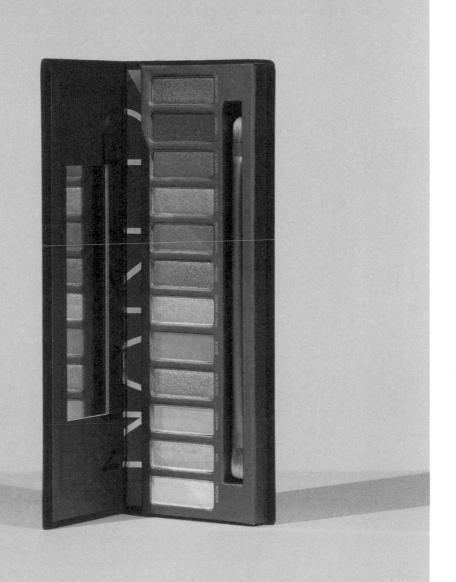

My relationship with the East Asian 'alphabet creams', as I refer collectively to BBs (Beauty or Blemish Balms), CCs (Colour Correcting), DDs (Daily Defence – milking it a bit) and EEs (Even Effect or Extra Exfoliating – Lord, give me strength), has been a rocky one. Even at the height of their enormous popularity circa 2013, I simply could not see what any of them offered that wasn't already being delivered far more attractively and effectively by a good tinted moisturiser and broad-spectrum facial sunscreen. Almost every one of them left my skin dry and gave me the radiance and subtle glow of a clay tagine. It seemed like wilful gimmickry for the sake of marketing, albeit very successful; my finger, as it turned out, was not on the pulse of consumer desire.

But in this Korean-made product I finally found something to shout about. Frankly, it makes mincemeat of every other CC cream I've tried (and I've tested several dozen). It evens dark patches, sunspots and redness, covers light blemishes and gives the whole face a brighter, very natural-looking, glowy veil of healthy colour. It's wonderful on casual weekends and lunches with friends, acts as an excellent base for other make-up, and comes from good stock; its Erborian stablemates (BBs, cushion bases and masks) are also very good. Its only significant fault is that it's suitable only for Caucasian and some Asian skin tones (for darker skins, I'd bypass the alphabet altogether and proceed directly to Nars Pure Radiant Tinted Moisturizer). I'm afraid that now, when Korean cosmetics have rightly entered the global mainstream, there is simply no longer some implicit excuse for Asian brands not to be racially inclusive (especially in this case, where Erborian is owned by L'Occitane). Buck up and make some deeper shades please, pronto.

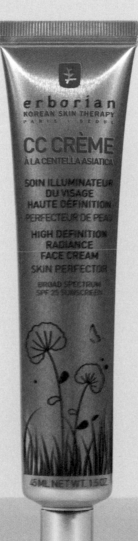

I love facialist Kate Somerville's skincare range. The ExfoliKate® (see what she did there?) scrub (a dead ringer for mint choc chip ice cream) is particularly good – if a little brutal for the unseasoned scrubber. Her Quench facial serum is among my all-time favourites, and I wouldn't be without her Clinic-To-Go® Resurfacing Peel Pads – little finger puppet pads of exfoliating acids that give tremendous glow and tell gaping pores to shut their mouths. But her most iconic offering is Goat Milk Moisturizing Cream, an elegant skin softener for dry and sensitive skins that I've adored since the first time I tried it upon launch into Space NK.

The cream hit the shelves in 2007 and first became a cult hit in the Pacific Northwest, where the cold and rain mean much dry and sensitive skin.

Other than its eponymous ingredient (which the young Somerville, who grew up on a farm, would have in her bath to counter the effects of severe eczema), the moisturiser sports a blend of reliable and unfaddy ingredients including witch hazel as well as sunflower, avocado, coconut, jojoba and grape oils.

The result is an extremely softening, gentle, luxury (read: expensive) moisturiser with impressive staying power. It's rich and satisfying and in my experience doesn't irritate. Those with acne or sensitive skin may get pleasing results too (I also find this and Elemis's Nourishing Milk Bath to be ideal presents for friends undergoing chemo who are in need of a fancy, but gentle, skin treat). The cream comes in a perfectly conceived and designed pump-action pot, which is airtight, preventing it from spoiling or the ingredients becoming destabilised. It should be the default packaging for creams everywhere.

The other good news is that after a period of unavailability in Britain, Kate Somerville – bought by Unilever in 2015 – will soon be returning to UK stores, but until then, these products can be bought and shipped internationally from Sephora.

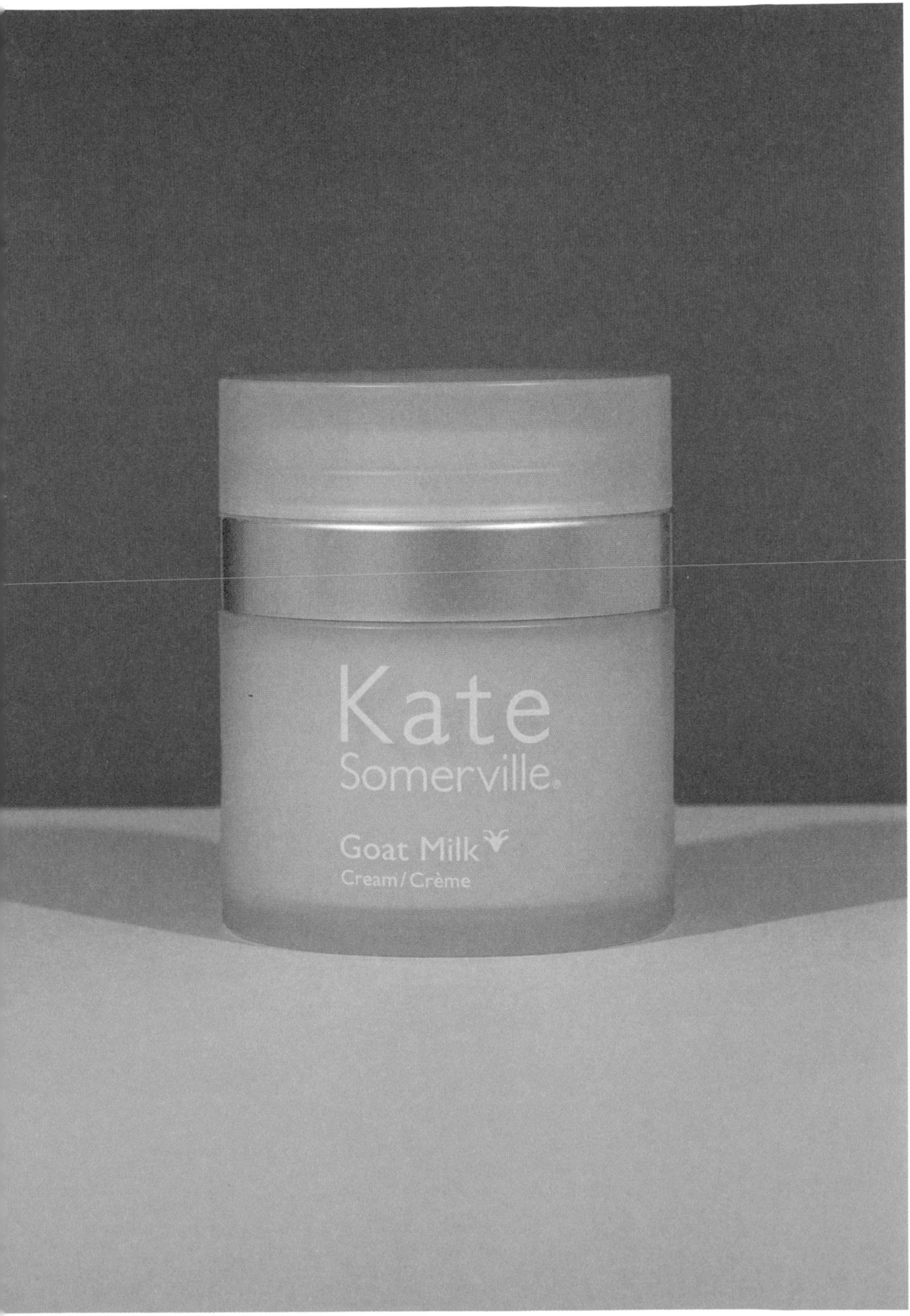
Kate
Somerville
Goat Milk
Cream/Crème

Just look at them. They're beautiful, aren't they? And sometimes that is more than enough. But for the avoidance of a blank page, I'll elaborate.

Lipstick fanatic Poppy King made her name in the 1990s, when the then-teenage Melburnian's eponymous, deadly sin-themed lipstick range became a multimillion-dollar success. King, though, was not one to rest on her laurels and after a spell working for Estée Lauder in New York she returned in 2006 with the Lipstick Queen line.

I'm so pleased she did, because these lipsticks are just beautiful. You can pluck one from your bag in any public place and immediately feel like a million dollars. They're weighty and tactile, classy and elegant, but still playful. The cases look like little art deco skyscrapers and belong in a satin-lined clutch with a silver cigarette case and dress gloves. The high-shine casing can double as a mirror – the magnetic closure snaps the lid into exactly the right position. These little details matter in luxury products, much as the click on a Bentley's glove-box door matters. Now, sometimes I'll mention a product's covetable packaging in a review and a reader will get cross, as though there's more merit in ignoring appearances and focusing only on the product within. I want to tell them that by the time you're talking about anti-ageing serums, sparkly nail polish and powder compacts, that particular principle has long since died a death. Appearances matter, and besides, packaging is important. I don't just mean the choice of font on the label, I'm talking about the way the whole thing is put together, the product delivery system, the method of ingress. If I don't enjoy using a product, if I find it fiddly or inconvenient, then I might just give up.

Don't think, though, that I'm laying the ground to tell you that Velvet Rope (the gold tubes containing matte lipstick) and Silver Screen (silver with a satin-finish lipstick) fail to live up to their first impressions. Not a bit of it. The super-saturated colours and luxurious-feeling formulas are so consistent I actually tend to take them for granted from King, like the dreadful parent of the school swot who regards a string of A* results as a given.

Needless to say, the lipsticks do not come cheap, and I personally feel it's reasonable to expect them to be refillable, which they aren't. The only other note of caution – do take them out of your bag at least five minutes before you plan to apply. It's nothing to do with the formula, it's just so you can stare at them for a bit.

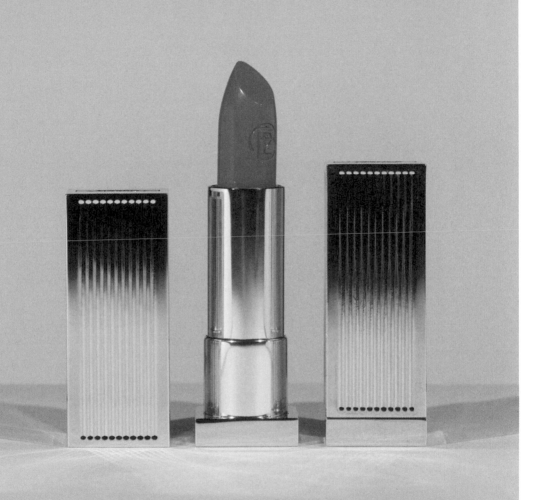

A brief riffle through this book will show that it features iconic, innovative beauty products that run the full gamut of technical intricacy. At one end of the scale, formulas of great chemical complexity, painstakingly composed through years of hard scientific research. At the other: a pink egg.

The Beautyblender is the brainchild of Rea Ann Silva, a make-up artist who realised that the advent of high-definition TV was going to force her to up her game. In order to create a look that would prove flawlessly line-free under the cameras' unforgiving gaze, she began to cut up sponges in her trailer, creating ellipses and spheres that allowed her to seamlessly blend make-up into every crease and contour of the face.

The fuchsia, ovoid Beautyblender was the result. It's a product that became absolutely huge almost entirely thanks to social media, where legions of bloggers, celebrities and make-up artists employed it to demonstrate their considerable and variable contouring techniques in countless video tutorials.

Beautyblender's technique is unique but straightforward. Apply make-up to your face, wet the sponge, it swells, then bounce the sponge off the face to blend in. This bouncing motion is essential as it allows the make-up to feather out without spreading elsewhere. And this is why contouring fanatics love it – stripes of colour stay resolutely in the contour lines, but soften around the edges for a more realistic-looking shadow (although 'realistic' in this context is very much a relative term). The Beautyblender absorbs less make-up than many others (hooray for that), and is reusable, which means less waste. A reusable sponge, it should go without saying, in turn means thorough cleaning – a stinky sponge is bad news for your skin.

The brand keeps reinventing the wheel to increase the business, including a white version for applying skincare (ridiculous and unhygienic. Why would you use a sponge when hands are invariably kept cleaner?), a 'red carpet' version (it's just red), a black 'pro' version (to avoid staining) and tiny versions that fall out of any non-Lilliputian hands. But the original is basically all you need and it's very good.

I must confess that I generally hate sponges and have done since I had to use upwards of thirty disposable wedges a day on pop video sets. From where I'm sitting, there's little a sponge can do that can't be done with a MAC duo-fibre brush. But I know I'm very much in the minority and besides, I fully believe the Beautyblender deserves props for identifying a global opportunity and totally owning it. If anything sums up beauty in 2016, it's the pink egg.

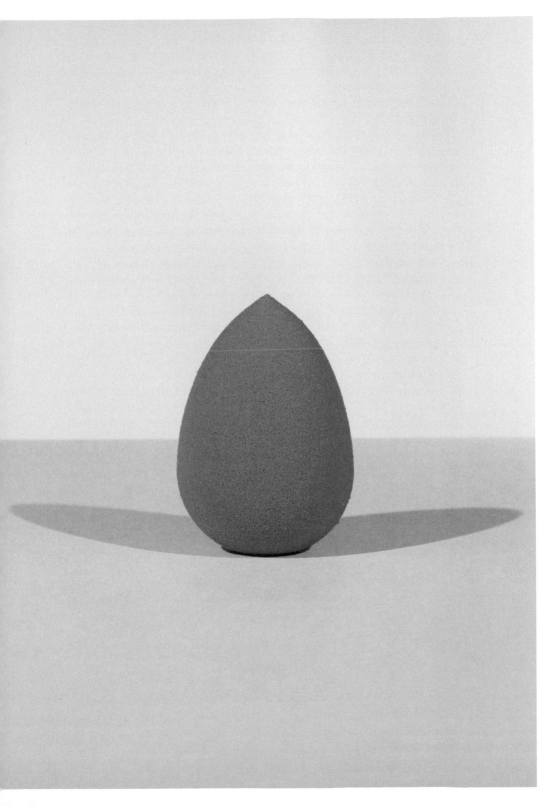

You're right, Perricone MD does sound like the kind of sub-Quincy detective series you might have watched from under a blanket on the sofa while off school, poorly. In fact, Dr Nicholas Perricone is the Connecticut dermatologist whose significance goes beyond any particular product in his big-selling skincare range. Perricone MD was perhaps the first success story in the field of cosmeceuticals.

Cosmeceuticals, as the name suggests, fall somewhere between traditional cosmetics and pharmaceutical products. Their origins lie in the offices of dermatologists, who can prescribe topical treatments containing a bigger whack of active ingredients than their clients would be able to get in an over-the-counter product. Enterprising professionals like Dr Perricone saw the opportunity to launch their own lines of product into the retail sector, the whiff of prescription-strength efficacy giving these treatments an edge over rival products from the traditional cosmetic giants. There's a degree of smoke and mirrors about all this: in law, there's no such thing as a cosmeceutical. If it's medication, it needs (in the USA) to be approved by the US Food and Drug Administration. If it's a cosmetic and sold in a store, it needn't. So for doctors to retail their product lines they often launch them with lower concentrations of the active ingredient in order to get under the regulation bar. Customers get the name, but not necessarily the prescription punch they were expecting.

In the case of Perricone's Cold Plasma range – the line of which the good doctor himself claims to be most proud – the company claimed to offer a new delivery system to get nutrients where the face needed them most, and that the product could effectively read your skin cells, only delivering those nutrients specifically required at the time. Whether you're a sceptic or confirmed Perriconista (and no, I didn't make that up), it's hard to deny that Dr Perricone changed the whole tone of cosmetics marketing. Where once product and packaging alike were all about prettiness, cosmeceuticals introduced the quasi-medical to the department store shelf, replacing dainty bottles with pipettes and functional dispensers, elegant labels with professional austerity and, in the case of most Perricone treatments I've encountered, a pleasant fragrance with the pong of rotten fish. The logic being, presumably, that anything that smelled this awful had to work.

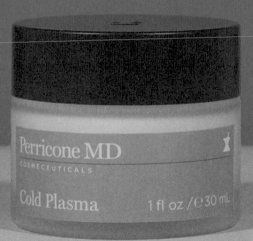

I first heard of airbrushing in 2000, when I attended a colour launch at Clinique, hosted by TV make-up artist Robin Siegel, best known as chief make-up designer on *Friends*. She had recently done Jennifer Aniston's make-up for her wedding to Brad Pitt and every journalist present was desperately (and quite rightly) trying to get the lowdown on the nuptials without appearing tacky or blowing their cover. It was perfectly obvious that Siegel was a class act and wasn't going to crack and so when it came to my turn, I asked her instead how she made the six actors' complexions so perfect on screen.

Airbrushing, was the answer. Siegel told me that since the advent of HD television, she had switched exclusively to water-based foundation sprayed onto the skin in a mist with a specialist electric airbrush. She was evangelical about it, explaining that her technique guaranteed no brush marks, no imperfections, no caking under the studio lights. I looked into getting one that week – not because I was about to try to break into showbiz, but because I can never bear not knowing what the fuss around a product is all about – and found they were about a grand in professional film make-up stores, so tried to forget the whole thing.

Some ten years later, I began doing the paper review on Sky News. As I sat in the make-up chair and the artist began to prepare a gun as though ready to spray the side of a pranged Volkswagen, I realised I'd finally got my chance. It was an important reminder that what looks great on camera (and it did) is not necessarily what looks good in real life (contouring fanatics take note), because, while my skin looked unusually great on camera, in the flesh it looked rather lifeless and flat, as though my features had melded into one. On my hands and lower arms (airbrushing is perfect for larger areas, since it works similarly to a spray tan) it was miraculous but, again, the price and size put me off and so I returned to the brilliant Scott Barnes Body Bling and James Read Wash Off Tan for summer and telly use.

My curiosity was finally rewarded with Temptu, launched in the UK via Space NK in 2016. Temptu – the market leaders in airbrushing – had scaled down their professional compressor and airbrush to a small domestic-use wand with clip-on pods of foundation, bronzer, highlighter and blush (they have since, rather ingeniously, begun selling hair root touch-up pods too). And I remain deeply impressed. I'm not sure whether airbrushing has got more subtle, or mainstream make-up has become so insanely obvious and mask-like, but the Temptu formulas are feather-light and extremely natural-looking, even when layered repeatedly to conceal broken veins or birthmarks, or when contouring (no obvious stripes here). The technique – wand held six inches away from the face and moved in small circles – is incredibly easy to master.

Apart from easy, airbrushing is also deeply satisfying. To say I got carried away on the first night would be an understatement. After I'd applied my eighth layer of make-up and officially run out of skin, I moved on to my assistant, then boyfriend. Had the dog not been sleeping and the kids already bathed, there's every chance I'd have sprayed them too. Oh and in case you were wondering – while I was ostensibly fascinated by Robin Siegel's love of airbrushing, I got her to admit that Jennifer was airbrushed for her wedding day. Journalism first.

It's a strange quirk of modern beauty that even as we complain about having less time to spend on our regime, we're embracing face masks more than ever. Until about 2010, masks were pretty much the preserve of the committed beauty nerd. To the less hardcore, they were something you might get during a facial or a spa weekend, or once in a blue moon when a last-minute cancellation left you and your face at a loose end on a Friday night.

Now it seems like masks are everywhere. I get sent so many new jars of clay I could build an extension out of the contents. I suspect selfie culture is at least in part to blame. Rather than do the grunt work of proper daily cleansing, toning and moisturising, people want perfect skin in fifteen minutes.

GlamGlow epitomises the trend as it's primarily about appearance rather than skin health. It came about when founders Glenn and Shannon Dellimore were entertaining actor friends in their house in the Hollywood Hills. So far, so relatable. Anyway, one thesp complained that no cosmetic would leave his skin instantly camera-ready, and Glenn and Shannon set about solving the problem. GlamGlow was the result. The range parades proprietary technologies and trademarks like Teaoxi, Acnecidic-6, Pore-Matrix, K17-Clay, Dewdration, Nitroffeine, Juvelane, Oilixier, Claytox and the brilliantly named Tapwipe, which sounds more like something you'd find in the Screwfix catalogue. Whether you suspect these pseudo-scientific portmanteau terms are compliballs, or buy into the dazzle like legions of faithful Glamaholics (they've even trademarked that, though personally I'd've gone for GlamGlow Rangers), there's no denying GlamGlow (bought by Estée Lauder a couple of years ago) has become a cult hit. Instant gratification sells.

Much as I love natural ingredients in beauty products, I'm no enemy of science. It's not like you'll find me turning up my nose at anything lab-manufactured just to smugly kick back with a homemade fox milk and ragwort face mask. I am decidedly pro chemicals and synthetics if they get the job done best, but for me, many of the very best beauty products are those that have most adroitly brought together science *and* nature. Sunday Riley's ethos is much the same. Riley studied chemistry at university in Texas, going on to work in cosmetics labs before launching her own line in 2009. Her timing was good. Thanks to a general backlash against synthetics and parabens (preservatives, present in most of our foods and many of our beauty products, which I personally believe to be utterly fine), plus the Internet and its more diverse beauty coverage creating a better understanding of skincare, facial oils were beginning to show signs of a revival and Riley was passionate about making them.

Having once been given a wide berth, oils have now become a huge part of the beauty industry. And while there is still a school of thought that's very anti these products, I'm a firm believer in the benefits of the right essential oils for your skin. A facial oil is an impatient girl's best friend. Unlike the kind of skincare that involves a lot of methodical application, patience and vigilance in order to see any benefit, an oil applied with a firm massage tonight will make you look better tomorrow than you did today. When I'm run down, tired or hungover, nothing else will do.

Sunday Riley's Hydroactive Cellular oil range is, almost without exception, very good indeed – though the pungent natural aromas are not to everyone's taste. I love the glow I get from Artemis (smell: school pencil shavings and lemon peel, designed for oily skins but oddly wonderful on my dry complexion); you may get better results from Juno (broccoli in a mud bath, for normal to dry) or Flora (spicy chicken, for dehydrated and super-dry skin. Previously named Isis. Probably best that's changed). I'm less convinced about Luna, Riley's blue retinol oil, but there are thousands of women who strongly disagree. I keep all of them in my bathroom, next to Riley's cruelly discontinued Stimulant Stem Cell Serum, the most instantly effective anti-ageing serum I have ever used in my life, which was torn away from me almost as soon as we met and is now reserved for occasions of critical importance.

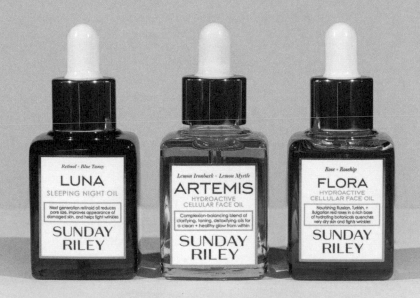

Vichy Aqualia Thermal Serum

In June 2014 I was having coffee and a catch up with a PR when she handed me a Vichy bottle, telling me it was 'just a new hydrating serum' but that I might like it. For me, someone with often woefully dehydrated skin, there is no such thing as 'just a new hydrating serum' – I try every single one that comes my way, without fail (not least because their effects are suitably immediate, making them quick to test). What especially intrigued me about this one was that it was by Vichy – a mid-price high street brand, rather than some super-expensive luxury label accessible only to a few. It has, I believe, taken an incredibly long time for high street brands in particular (though not exclusively) to come around to the fact that dry and dehydrated mean very different things, even when they come as a pair (today, as I write, I have tested two high street products and one luxury, all of them for dehydration, and I wouldn't recommend you spend even tuppence of your hard-earned cash on any of them). The simple explanation is this: dry skin lacks oil, dehydrated skin lacks water. Dry skin therefore craves rich creams, oils and other emollients, while dehydrated skins benefit hugely from humectants like glycerin, and the presence of hyaluronic acid, a substance naturally present in the body, which has the ability to hold around a thousand times its weight in water. A really good hydration serum cannot create water from nowhere, but it can cling on to what's there and refuse to let go all day, giving skin a plumper, less crêpey, more comfortable and smooth surface.

Within six hours of receiving my sample, I believed that Vichy Aqualia Thermal serum did this better than any other hydration serum under £25. I began using it regularly, choosing it over some serums costing five times as much. It's the serum that lives permanently in my travel vanity case because it always works; it's the serum I consistently reach the end of and have to take out the pump and slam it hard against my palm, like a sluggish ketchup bottle. One could reasonably accuse me of having banged on about Vichy Aqualia to the point of tedium, but there are countless readers who tell me frequently that their now better-hydrated skin thanks me for it. And while I wouldn't normally take the credit for the increased popularity of a single product (it's generally much more the result of a cumulative buzz than of one person raving about something – if the latter were true, Dior would never have discontinued Glow Maximiser primer, damn it), in the case of Vichy Aqualia and (the also very good) Superdrug Simply Pure Hydrating Serum, I think I justifiably can.

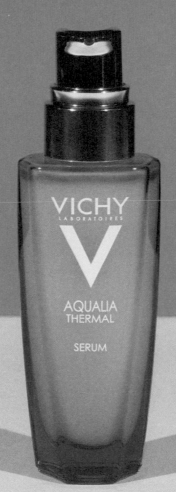

I could no more name my single favourite lipstick than I could pick a favourite Beatles' song. I have previously tried but before I know it I have a shortlist of mattes: MAC Lady Danger, Nars Heat Wave and Rosecliff; semi-mattes: Charlotte Tilbury Stoned Rose and Bitch Perfect, Estée Pure Color Envy in Insatiable Ivory, Rebellious Rose and Envious, Burberry Rosewood and Military Red; satins: Bobbi Brown Nude, Chanel's Rouge Coco in Mademoiselle and (my son's namesake) Arthur; sheers: Tom Ford Nubile and Frolic, Poppy King Lipstick Queen's Medieval, Clinique's Black Honey, Surratt's Lipslique in Bandy. Add a fleet of seasonal flings and the shortlist resembles the Magna Carta.

But if I had to put forward an entire collection, on the basis of the collective brilliance of its formula, packaging, colour range, finish and application, I'd choose Nars Audacious. This range of lipsticks, launched in 2014, is as close as I've seen to across the board perfection. The formula is dense, opaque, lasting and bold but comes at no cost to comfort (so many drag and dry). There is not a single dud among the colours; from classic to edgy, nude to dramatic (Lana, a vintage-looking *Mad Men* orange-red, is glorious). They are perfectly curated without glitter, shimmer or frost. The finish is ideal for my taste – almost matte but with a fraction of slip to allow light to catch flatteringly on the mouth. The packaging is cool, stylish satiny black metal, tactile but sturdy with an unshowy black logo. It is a perfect lipstick. And I don't say that lightly. But before the extremely charming Monsieur Nars kicks back on his private island, believing his work here is done, I should say that I will never, ever stop looking for something better.

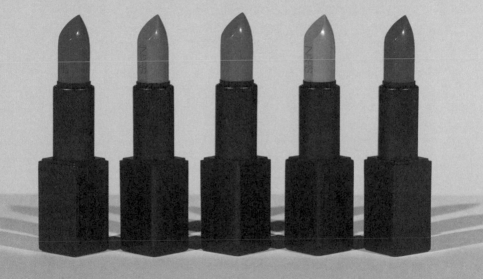

When I first moved to London in 1990, the make-up artist population would have been somewhere in the region of two to three dozen, each of them working regularly and employing make-up assistants thanks to decent production budgets, more extras on set and a thriving fashion and music industry. So I feel extremely lucky to have walked into a Soho bar when I did, to have been introduced to make-up artist Lynne Easton, and to have been asked to be her assistant. Even ten, never mind twenty-six, years later, when social media has brought about nothing short of a revolution in make-up artistry, the competition would have been way too fierce.

On the one hand, I think it's wonderful. I love that the Internet has given so many men and women access to what can amount to the kind of professional training that was previously only available at a handful of colleges or on the job, that any talented artist with a smartphone can create her own content, showcase her skills and find an audience. It's exciting to be part of a huge and diverse community rather than the comparatively tiny cult I first joined. But on the other, I feel sorry for those trying to monetise their often considerable skills in this strapped and increasingly tight-fisted industry. Whereas I, at 15, was being paid £50–£80 a day to assist on shoots, now young artists are expected to work for nothing for years on end. Indie film and fashion companies demand free labour in order to balance their books, known make-up artists receive thousands of begging letters and emails from high-calibre wannabe assistants every year, and even those who make it through can find themselves doing little more than admin.

And so while I understand that beauty careers, like homeownership, must seem to have been so much easier then than now, allow me to offer aspiring artists a small crumb of comfort: your kit is so, so much cheaper, and better, than ours. My first professional kit contained cheap paintbrushes from an art shop and a few CD cases, emptied and refilled with whatever crappy pans of old eyeshadow and blush I could prise from their packaging without cracking the powder inside. If I wanted a blendable matte eyeshadow (there was no MAC, and everything on the high street was frosty) I had to save my money to buy pans, one by one, from professional stockist Screenface. Empty palettes and high-quality brushes cost fortunes, and no affordable foundations existed in any colour but American tan and Band-Aid pink. The cost of building up a proper kit was frankly traumatic. I often think about this now, when I'm unpacking wonderful samples from Models Own, Rimmel London, Zoeva and Topshop, or when I'm browsing in Superdrug and see Real Techniques brushes, Makeup Revolution shadows and these, Sleek i-Divine palettes. From these brands alone, you could build up an entire kit way better than the one I worked with on commercials and pop videos – i-Divine eyeshadows in particular are a gamechanger for young professionals. There's no look that you can't achieve, no texture unavailable, no colour excluded. Like all Sleek formulas, the shadows are brilliant – blendable and long-lasting with stronger colour payoff than many at four times the price. The palettes themselves are slim, well put together and look professional to anyone passing the make-up room. If Sleek had existed when I started out, I'd have had a lot more make-up and eaten a whole lot less plain pasta.

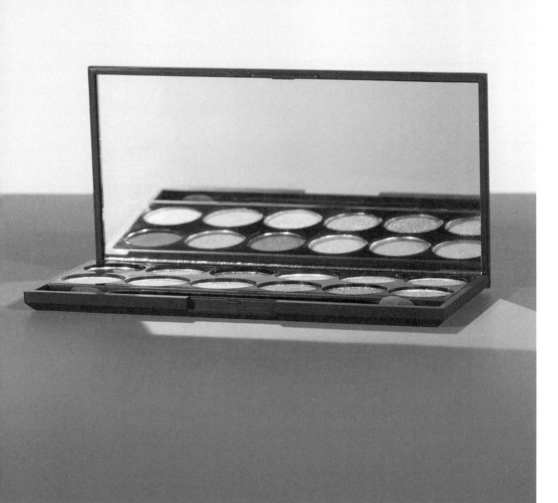

Toner and I have an uneasy, oft-misunderstood, relationship, so I should clarify (no pun intended). In summary: I think traditional toners, i.e. skin tonics or floral waters containing herbs, honey, roses, cucumber, chamomile or whatever it is a brand is claiming will 'remove the last traces of cleanser and tighten pores', are an utter nonsense. A nice nonsense, admittedly, and if you enjoy using toner then you absolutely should continue. But what I object to is the traditional default position adopted by brands that women must buy a toner in order to do skincare right. It is simply untrue and in twenty-five years, not one expert has ever been able to convince me otherwise. A hot, wrung-out flannel will remove all traces of cleanser and no toner has the power to tighten pores for any respectable period of time. Save your money or buy some wine and a book.

What I do believe in are liquid exfoliants, which are increasingly and confusingly now referred to by many as 'toners'. Liquid exfoliants are lotions containing either Alpha Hydroxy Acids (AHAs) or Beta Hydroxy Acids (BHAs) or both, and work by sloughing and sweeping away dead skin cells, leaving skin physically smoother and brighter in appearance; with the dead, dull layer gone, fine lines are minimised and light bounces off the healthy cells beneath. As a bonus, the skin is better prepared to accept more long-term skincare products.

Alpha-H did not invent the liquid exfoliant. Clinique has been selling them for decades and was the first to popularise liquid exfoliants back in the 1960s, and many have launched since (Dr Dennis Gross peel pads happen to be my usual weapon of choice). But when, in around 2008, liquid exfoliants began a huge twenty-first-century comeback, Alpha-H's 8-year-old Liquid Gold was at the forefront of the revival and, thanks to the Internet, developed a huge cult following without a great deal of editorial coverage (probably because of its deeply unalluring packaging and branding) or any advertising. The rise of the beauty blogger was key to its success.

Liquid Gold is not for everyone. Some folk are put off liquid exfoliants because they contain acids. It's an understandable instinct for the uninitiated, possibly picturing some kind of gothic chemistry lab horror in which a quick swipe of toner leaves nothing above the neck but a grimacing skull, but the acids here are of a nature and quantity that won't do anything really drastic. Having said that, Liquid Gold does have one of the higher concentrations of acids on the market (its featured ingredient is glycolic acid, one of the AHAs alongside citric and lactic acids that have great anti-ageing properties) and as such is not ideal for very sensitive skin. For the most part, though, even if acids irritate you at first, you can generally build up a tolerance by starting with a product with a much smaller concentration and letting your skin acclimatise. I'd also recommend applying at night as that lovely, newly-revealed skin may also be sensitive to strong sunlight, and even then, only twice a week.

The other cautionary note with Liquid Gold is that it contains alcohol, something I would generally swerve where possible. I must say, though, it seems fine here and doesn't cause extra dryness in my experience. Your mileage, of course, may vary, and while I'm a big fan of liquid exfoliants, Alpha-H's offering is perhaps one for the more hardened acidheads.

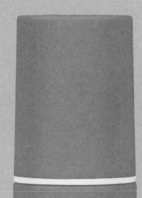

ALPHA-H

LIQUID GOLD™
WITH
GLYCOLIC ACID

100ml/3.38 fl.oz
COINCENTRATED SKINCARE

If I had to choose one product I believe in more than any other, just one that I'd want readers to go out and buy, use and say, 'Bloody hell, she was right!', I feel certain it would be the Boots Electronic Cold Sore Machine (previously 'Avert'). Barely a week goes by without a reader getting in touch with me to say this slightly crap-looking, seemingly lo-tech gadget has changed their life immeasurably, just as it has mine.

I got my first cold sore when I was 24. A man I barely knew leaned in to peck me on the cheek before I could identify that he had a huge, weeping sore on his mouth. And that was that. What lay ahead was ten years of (mercifully intermittent) misery. Whenever I caught a cold, I knew the hangover would come in the form of a cold sore (I've come to believe, as many do, that my cold or flu symptoms *are* the cold sore, not the cause of one). As soon as the sun came out for summer, I got a cold sore. Every February, without fail, I got a cold sore for my birthday.

Then one day, as I was writing my column in a café, trying not to speak to the waiter for fear of my gigantic cold sore cracking painfully and bleeding, a Google search led me to Avert. I went out immediately and bought one, zapped the sore as directed and within two hours all the swelling around my mouth had gone. The next day, the sore had scabbed over. I kept zapping. Within four days, it was gone – a good ten days ahead of the usual schedule.

Now, as soon as I feel a sore throat developing, or feel the dreaded tingle on my mouth, I grab one of my two Avert machines (one lives next to my bed, the other in my handbag – to be caught short is maddening), place it over my mouth, press the button and hold it there for the full four minutes until the Avert beeps to tell me the treatment (using light therapy) is complete. I do this three to four times a day thereafter (the box says twice is sufficient but I am a somewhat unrestrained person by nature). Even if the cold sore does still appear, it tends to be puny, not the classic weeping, agonising, bleeding, throbbing, size-of-a-Ford-Mondeo sore I suffered for many years. It'll resemble an untroubling zit and be safely confined to the lip itself, not invading the upper area. It will be completely sealed and not weeping at all. There'll be no scab, no pain or even discomfort and no one else in the house will even notice it's there.

But this is highly unlikely. Because the truly remarkable thing is that thanks to using Avert pre-emptively a couple of times a week since I bought it, I've had a grand total of four cold sores in five years. FIVE YEARS. That is five years of not feeling ill, cancelling engagements you've been looking forward to for months, too paranoid that you'll unwittingly infect someone, too self-conscious about the throbbing Wotsit attached to your upper lip. Five years of having conversations with your hands at your side, not covering your lower face as though your companion has noxious halitosis. Five years of being able to kiss your children whenever they want you to, of not throwing good money at super-expensive creams that don't work. Cold sores are dreadful. This is a miracle. Go and get one.

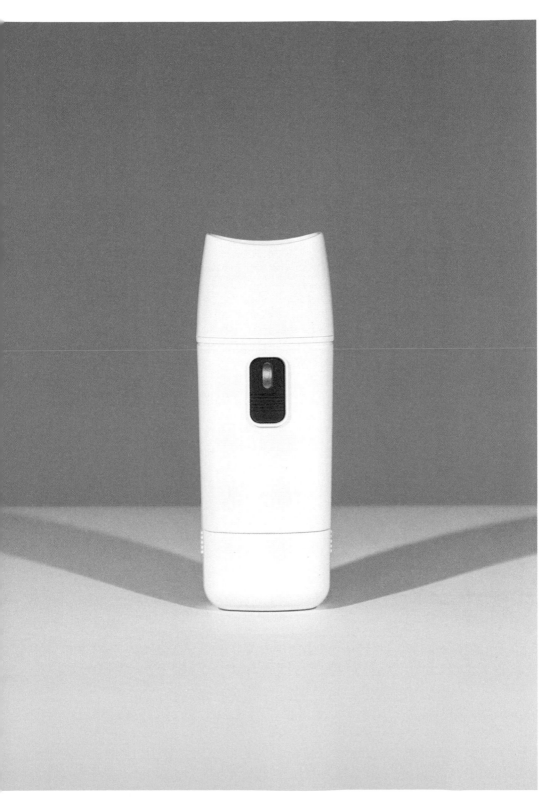

This perennial favourite can reputedly trace its ancestry back to the delicious-sounding Crème Céleste, an almond oil and rose water concoction used by the nineteenth-century Empress Elisabeth of Austria-Hungary.

There's nothing aristocratic or remotely high-and-mighty about its 1967 descendant, though, which is a lovely, unpretentious day cream. Like an understanding best friend, Rose Day Cream is there waiting for me when a liaison with a harsh product I'm testing has left my skin suffering. It's simple and soothing and there's nothing showy in it. Or on the outside, for that matter: I love its unassuming packaging, which is surely in contention for design classic status and somehow manages to make brown-rice-and-sandals austerity seem quite desirable (I always think of its orange and white design as the Penguin Classics book jacket of beauty). The fact that Kate Moss apparently loves the stuff probably helps too, in all honesty.

The cream's floral extracts help to keep the skin balanced; avocado oil, shea butter and rose petal wax moisturise and the soothing quality comes from extracts of St John's wort and marshmallow (yes, the plant. Sadly they don't boil down the treats). It is not ideally suited to oily or highly sensitive skins (I acknowledge that there is a movement against plant oils, though I'm certainly no part of it), but normal and dry types should like it.

It's also lovely as a make-up base, and thankfully comes in tubes. I do wish the beauty industry would stop assuming we want everything in jars. They really are the most impractical, unhygienic and scientifically unsound way to store active ingredients and are good for little more than peanut butter.

01.2018

Dr. Hauschka

Rosen
Tagescreme

Rose
Day Cream

I love Charlotte Tilbury for many reasons. Obviously, she's a brilliant make-up artist – among the finest we've ever seen. Her talent, eye for faces and sense of glamour are innate. She delights in making normal women look like goddesses and her passion for beauty is infectious.

But what I personally love just as much is that Tilbury is a grafter. She didn't emerge fully-formed from a lofty, wafty, heritage beauty house but worked her way up, starting out as an assistant and steadily building a network of photographers, stylists and models as she went, until she was fully established at the top table, world renowned and, in 2013, ready to launch her own brand. She believes in her product and markets it with considerable moxie and commercial nous. To host a public event with Charlotte – as I have on a few occasions – is invariably to see her end up on her 6-inch heels, handbag opened hastily on the floor, pulling out a product and lovingly applying it to the faces of audience members, then making absolutely sure they know where to go and buy it. The approach is charming and, it must be said, very much in the admirable hands-on, old-school, hard-selling tradition of beauty mavens Mrs Lauder, Arden and Rubinstein.

Rather than sell bits of product individually and shorn of context, Charlotte Tilbury's thing is to market make-up in complete 'faces': the Sophisticate, the Uptown Girl, the Ingénue and so on, with an eyeshadow quad at the heart of each look. This canny approach helps sell multiple items across the range and has had a lot to do with the brand's almost unprecedented success.

All this interests me, but as a beauty writer, the most commendable aspect of the launch of Tilbury's brand was that she and her business partner, Demetra Pinsent, put all their money not into advertising, marketing or fancy packaging, but into getting the product right.

The best example of this attention to formula is in the aforementioned eye palettes (though I love the blushers, brushes, pencils and pressed powder almost as much). These shadows are brilliant – a combination of matte, satin and shimmer, arranged and labelled logically to achieve different effects. The shades are superbly blendable, the colour payoff great. And speaking only for myself here, I need no more than four shades in a case – I loathe waste and any more just begs for shadows to go unused.

These are, she may not thank me for saying, not a million miles from the beautiful eye palettes by Tom Ford, a brand with which Tilbury was once closely associated. But for me these edge it as they are handbag-friendly, more affordable, don't waste space with daft applicators, and walk women through an entire look. The Sophisticate is my go-to neutral palette for work meetings, while Golden Goddess, Rock Chick or the Rebel all give different nuances to nighttime. And they are genuinely easy. Despite the fact that much is made of Tilbury's A-list and supermodel connections, her personal mission statement is to make every woman look like the most beautiful version of themselves. And if she can build a multi-million pound empire while doing it, then that's *just gorgeous, darling.*

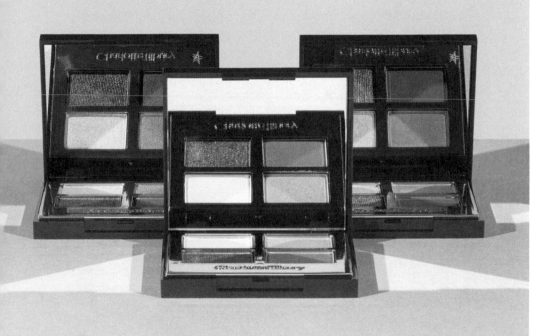

In 2002 I was working on *ELLEgirl* magazine, alongside the extremely talented fashion editor, Steph Stevens (now noted for her work with Alexa Chung and *Stella* magazine). One day, Steph walked into the office smelling so delicious I could have swallowed her whole. Diptyque's Philosykos was the answer to my inevitable question, and so with her permission and my assurances that I wouldn't wear it at work (there's nothing worse than having someone claim your signature scent), off I went at lunchtime to buy my own bottle of liquid fresh fig. I loved Philosykos deeply and instantly and many years later I realise it might be only one of about five perfumes I've replaced repeatedly when empty (the bulk of my scent collection evolves like a little black book of suitors – only a handful are marriage material), and is easily the most admired.

Whenever I wear it, someone is guaranteed to remark on how unusual it is, how comforting yet wholly unfamiliar at the same time. Philosykos may no longer be as unique as when I discovered it – nowadays, figgy scents are everywhere, often synthetic, too tart, and a sort of default choice for people who say they don't much like perfume. But Philosykos itself remains extraordinary, and is by far and away the best of them: ripe, fresh, as gorgeous on a man as on a woman (no one does unisex as naturally and as unfussily as Diptyque), a shot of sour green and mossy wood sap to stem the stickiness of the fruit.

Memorably – given that experience has shown me that Philosykos is, by some distance, the scent most likely to elicit compliments and the least likely to be identified – I once met a fellow writer at a Christmas lunch who, having politely kissed me hello, asked me if I was wearing Diptyque Philosykos. Impressed, I asked how he knew, wondering if he wore it too. He said he just had a thing for killing the odd hour between meetings in the Liberty perfumery, testing fragrances, collecting blotter strips and making a mental note of those he liked, Philosykos being one of them and L'Ombre dans l'Eau, the beautiful rose and blackcurrant scent he was wearing, being another.

And so we began a lengthy conversation about our favourite perfumes and smells, the best scented candles (he: Cire Trudon and English Eccentrics; me: Miller Harris and Diptyque), why he was entirely wrong about Cacharel's Loulou being an abomination but oh so right about Chanel's Pour Monsieur being glorious. And while Philosykos can't claim to be the longest lasting perfume, it did hold its own and remain present for most of the hours of happy chat that followed, until I went home, feeling delighted to have made a new friend, thinking how joyful it is to talk products with a man who seems to understand and appreciate my level of nerdery, if not entirely share it.

Reader, I did not marry him. But we do live very happily in sin.

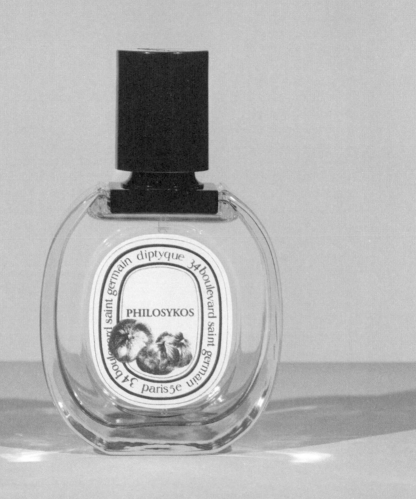

Acknowledgements

First and foremost, thank you to the always sane, calm and considered Georgia Garrett at RCW: it's beyond a joke how good an agent you are. Thank you also to Louise Haines and her wonderful, hard-working team, who immediately understood this slightly odd book, just as they had the last, and were beyond patient when I realised gradually how hard it would be. I feel honoured to be part of the 4th Estate family. Big thanks also to another of its members, Nigel Slater, who quite unwittingly inspired both my choice of publisher and the theme of this book. Thank you also to Morag Lyall for her eagle-eyed fact-checking and copy editing, Sam Wolfson for another clever design, and to my dear friend Jake Walters for the unwavering calm, professionalism and beautiful photography.

I'm forever grateful to my assistant Lauren Oakey, who contacted every existing brand in the book, begging for dates and sales figures, pleading for picture rights and archive imagery, keeping her cool when many brands either ignored or dismissed her or tried to pay their way into the book (yes, really) – all while being way too young to even remember Constance Carroll or Toni perms. Similarly, I am indebted to the small number of PRs and brands who trusted me enough to go hugely out of their way for a book I wouldn't fully describe for them. Extra special thanks to Nathalie Everard at Chanel, Jo Jones at TCS, Mel Jones at Estée Lauder, Terry Barber for the drunken product reminiscing, Sam McKnight for the late night Carmen and Magic Move chats, and to the endlessly kind, clever and generous Mary Greenwell.

My day job editors and colleagues, as ever, have been very supportive during the book writing process. Enormous thanks to Debra Brock of salihughesbeauty.com, whom we both know I really don't deserve, to Nat Saunders for being In the Bathroom with me from the very beginning, and to all the wonderful admins, moderators and members who make the forum such a special place. Thank you also to Sam Baker and Lauren Laverne of the-pool.com and to Terri White of *Empire*, three beloved friends I'm proud to call my bosses, and to the extremely patient and long-suffering Hannah Marriott at the *Guardian* – a paper that never, ever asks me to scratch any backs, nor do any favours. A rare thing indeed.

Thanks to Marian Keyes for All of the Things, to my fellow beauty junkie and childhood friend Brigette Hughes, the first person I turned to in order to jog my memory, to Cathy Rentzenbrink, whose wine-fuelled chats kept me sane during our week's 'writing retreat' in a Stroud cottage, as well as to Alice Lowe for letting us stay there. And especially to Bryony Gordon for talking me down from the ledge, and India Knight for her peerless hostessing skills during the thick end of this book. Thank you to the rest of my friends, without whom I would go completely 'shoebag': you all know exactly who you are.

Finally, my unending gratitude to live-in nag Daniel Maier, whose love, support and encouragement have been unwavering and frankly life-changing. My good fortune is extraordinary, and I could do nothing without you, least of all write a book. And to my darling Marvin and Arthur, who I'm glad will no longer be asking 'How many words are left?', but who remain the primary reason I do anything and everything. I love all of you more than lipstick. xx

Picture Credits

Permission to use archive material kindly provided by:

Max Factor Creme Puff – Image Courtesy of The Advertising Archives;
Mason Pearson Hairbrushes – Early POS advertising for Mason Pearson
  hairbrushes, with thanks to Mason Pearson;
Max Factor Pan-Cake – Image Courtesy of The Advertising Archives;
Erno Laszlo – Image Courtesy of The Advertising Archives;
Avon Ladies – Image Courtesy of The Advertising Archives;
Coppertone – Image Courtesy of The Advertising Archives;
Dove Campaign for Real Beauty – Image Courtesy of The Advertising Archives;
Revlon Charlie – Image Courtesy of The Advertising Archives;
The Boots Christmas Gift Catalogue 1981 – Boots UK Archives.

Additional thanks to GF Smith for their papers in the photographs.